260 ESSENTIAL ·CHINESE· MEDICINALS

本草

二百六十主要中草药

BY

Bob Flaws

BLUE • POPPY • PRESS

Published by:

Blue Poppy Press
A Division of Blue Poppy Enterprises, Inc.
3450 Penrose Place, Suite 110
Boulder, CO 80301
(303) 447-8372

First Edition March, 1999

ISBN 1-891845-03-9
Library of congress Catalog Card #98-74794

COMP Designation: Original work

Printed at Johnson Printing
Cover design by Anne Rue

10, 9, 8, 7, 6, 5, 4, 3, 2 , 1

Preface

For many years, I assumed there was no need for me to compile a materia medica. Bensky & Gamble's *Chinese Herbal Medicine: Materia Medica* is the standard materia medica text used in English language schools of Chinese medicine worldwide. However, when I decided to teach a course in Chinese herbal medicine, I realized that I could not use that text since it uses a different translational terminology than the one I and Blue Poppy Press endorse. Many of the problems Western students and practitioners have with the practice of Chinese medicine stem from using an inexact translational terminology. In Chinese, Chinese medicine is described with great technical precision. When the Chinese medical literature is translated into English, much of that technical precision is lost because the linguistic logic and connections inherent in the original Chinese are lost. Although I continue to believe that one must learn to read at least modern medical Chinese if one really wants to understand how to do Chinese medicine, I also believe that Nigel Wiseman's translational terminology as described in his *English-Chinese Chinese-English Dictionary of Chinese Medicine* preserves to the greatest degree possible in English to date the technical implications so often glossed over by other translational approaches. Therefore, once I decided that I would teach a course in Chinese herbal medicine, I was faced with having to create a materia medica using Wiseman's terminology.

My second purpose in compiling this materia medica was to create a smaller, cheaper materia medica which would be easier to carry around, study, and use than Bensky and Gamble's. I wanted to focus students' attention on the most important medicinals and most important information about those medicinals, while presenting this material in a nonetheless attractive, easy to read format.

This materia medica is the fruit of those desires. It primarily focuses on what I take to be the main 260 medicinals in the contemporary practice of Chinese medicine. Both Bensky and Gamble and Hong-yen Hsu's *Oriental Materia Medica: A Concise Guide* contain more individual ingredients and I recommend those two books as English language sources for those medicinals which did not make the cut into this book. In choosing which medicinals to include in this current work, I chose those which comprise the ingredients in the main standard formulas of Chinese medicine administered as water-based decoctions as well as those commonly found in Chinese prepared or patent medicines. I had originally intended to include fewer than the number of medicinals herein. However, once I got started, I was hard put to whittle the number any lower and still have this materia medica be representative of contemporary Chinese clinical practice. Students should know that the medicinals presented first in each chapter are the most important and commonly used.

This materia medica does contain ingredients from several endangered species, such as the rhinoceros and Saiga antelope. These ingredients can easily be substituted for by those from non-endangered species. Blue Poppy Press neither supports or endorses the use of endangered species in Chinese medicine, and we urge all our readers not to purchase or prescribe any medicines containing medicinals made from such endangered species. I have included medicinals from endangered species in this book so as to remain consistent to the Chinese medical tradition. But I most emphatically do not recommend or endorse their use.

Under each medicinal, the reader will find several categories of information. First is the medicinal's name given in Latin pharmacological nomenclature. This is followed in parentheses by the medicinal's most common Chinese name spelled in Pinyin romanization. Next comes the medicinal's nature and flavor. There are five natures: cold, cool, level or neutral, warm, and hot. There are six flavors: sweet, acrid, bitter, sour, salty, and bland. Slightly cold or slightly hot are the same as cool and warm respectively. In addition, some medicinals are listed as having small toxins or toxins. This is the same as saying that they are slightly toxic or toxic.

After nature and flavor, the next category of information on each medicinal is their channel entry. Although the term channel is used, the names following this heading are simply those of the five viscera and six bowels. These are the viscera and bowels upon which each medicinal exerts the greatest influence. This information is inferred based on the diseases and symptoms each medicinal is empirically known to treat and Chinese medicine's theory about the various viscera bowels' role in the disease mechanisms of these conditions and symptoms.

Channel entries are followed by functions. These are the Chinese medical actions of each medicinal stated in the same terminology as Chinese medical treatment principles. These functions tell one what each medicinal does theoretically. Correlated to these functions and based on empirical experience, one next sees each medicinal's clinical indications. These are a list of the main conditions treated by the medicinal as well as their most important and/or common combinations. While the functions tell the reader what the medicinal does in theory, the indications tell the reader what the medicinal does in fact. These two groups of information must be taken together before one can have a good Chinese medical idea of how a medicinal works and when to use it.

After indications come dosage. This is the contemporary standard daily dose when used as an ingredient in a water-based polypharmacy decoction in the People's Republic of China. If it refers to something other than that, such as the dose when taken as a pill or powder, this is specified as such. After dosage comes method of use. The most common method of use is to decoct in water and administer internally. This is also where specific instructions on cooking times or techniques for particular medicinals are given. In addition, information on processing prior to decoction is also given for a number of the most important medicinals used in processed forms.

And finally, after methods of use, comes cautions and contraindications. This category of information alerts the reader to any special cautions or contraindications that should be take when using a particular medicinal. Chinese medicinals are not *ipso facto* safe. They are only safe when they are administered in the right patient based on the right pattern discrimination and in the right dose for the right length of time. If a medicinal is powerful enough to bring a condition back to balance, then it must also be strong enough to throw the body out of balance if administered erroneously. There is no universal panacea!

In the actual day to day prescription of Chinese medicinals, I believe the functions and indications are the most important pieces of information to be kept in mind. The functions are related to the nature, flavor, and channel entry. However, there are many differences of opinion about these first three categories of information. Because the functions are stated in the same language as Chinese treatment principles and because the treatment principles are the bridge between the pattern discrimination and the actual treatment plan, I believe that the functions are vitally important and should be memorized as carefully as possible. In fact, I have created this materia medica largely to provide a framework for the presentation of each the main Chinese medicinals' functions in Nigel Wiseman's terminology. They are that important!

The information in this materia medica has been taken from a number of Chinese language sources. These are listed in the bibliography in the back. I hope this materia medica helps Western students more easily and accurately memorize the main medicinals of Chinese medicine. These medicinals are like the ABCs. They are the building blocks of Chinese medicinal formulas. Before one can understand how to prescribe and write Chinese medicinal formulas, one must have a firm foundation in the materia medica. In fact, one should *never* prescribe any ingredient of which one does not know the nature, flavor, functions, indications, dosage, and cautions and contraindications.

For more information on the development and history of the materia medica literature within Chinese medicine, the reader should see Paul U. Unschuld's *Medicine in China: A History of Pharmaceutics*. For a comparison of the modern Chinese materia medica literature as embodied in this text with an ancient Chinese materia medica, the reader should see *The Divine Farmer's Materia Medica*, a translation of the *locus classicus* of all Chinese materia medica, the *Shen Nong Ben Cao Jing*. For information on the interactions, both wanted and unwanted, between Chinese medicinals, please see Philippe Sionneau's *Dui Yao: The Art of Combining Chinese Medicinals*. For information on the methods of processing Chinese medicinals prior to their being used in decoction and on the functions and indications of differently processed Chinese medicinals, please see Sionneau's *Pao Zhi: An Introduction to the Use of Processed Chinese Medicinals*. For a repertoire of 70 essential Chinese medicinal formulas, the reader is directed to my *Seventy Essential TCM Formulas for Beginners*, while for a discussion of the step-by-step methodology of writing prescriptions and modifying Chinese medicinal formulas, see my

How to Write a TCM Herbal Formula. In addition, *The Heart Transmission of Medicine* is a translation of a Qing dynasty primer on the practice of medicine with an emphasis on the most important standard formulas within Chinese medicine and their modification to fit a large variety of patterns and conditions. If one had a good command of the information within these several books, this, armed with a basic understanding of Chinese medical theory and treatment based on pattern discrimination, would provide the basics of understanding the clinical practice of Chinese herbal medicine. For the key statements of fact which form the foundation of the theory of Chinese medicine, the reader should see my *Statements of Fact in Traditional Chinese Medicine.* For an in-depth discussion of treatment based on pattern discrimination and a compendium of all the main patterns currently used in Chinese medicine, see my *A Compendium of TCM Patterns & Treatments.* And finally, for explanations of the technical implications of the terms used in this book, please see Nigel Wiseman's *A Practical Dictionary of Chinese Medicine.* Bibliographic information on all these books is given in the bibliography at the rear of this book.

Bob Flaws
January 1999

Table of Contents

Exterior-resolving medicinals

Medicinals which mainly have the effect of effusing and scattering exterior evils and resolving and eliminating exterior patterns are called exterior-resolving medicinals. Such exterior-resolving medicinals are mostly acrid-flavored, windy-natured medicinals which are able to promote the scattering of external evils located in the muscular exterior via sweating. Thus they are suitable for use in external contraction conditions. Various of these medicinals also have the effects of diffusing the lungs, stopping coughing, leveling[1] asthma, out-thrusting rashes, disinhibiting urination, and dispersing swelling and hence can be used for non-diffusion of the lung qi coughing and panting, wind damp impediment pain, wind rash, measles, and water swelling.

Exterior-resolving medicinals are divided into two types: acrid and warm exterior-resolving medicinals and acrid and cool exterior-resolving medicinals. Acrid and warm exterior-resolving medicinals are used primarily in cases of wind cold exterior patterns, while acrid and cool exterior-resolving medicinals are used primarily in case of wind heat exterior patterns. Both groups of medicinals can be combined with other medicinals, such as those which transform phlegm, stop coughing, clear heat, move the qi, dispel dampness, or even supplementing and boosting medicinals, depending on the patient's pattern, presenting signs and symptoms, and bodily constitution.

When using this category of medicinals, the dosage should be just the right amount and their use should be stopped as soon as their use is no longer warranted. Otherwise, excessive perspiration can consume and scatter yang qi and cause detriment and damage to fluids and humors. These medicinals should be used cautiously or are contraindicated in case of exterior vacuity spontaneous perspiration, yin vacuity fever, the latter stages of warm diseases with fluid and humor depletion and consumption, loss of blood, enduring sores and welling abscesses, and strangury conditions. Depending on the environment and the seasonal qi, their dose should be increased or decreased. Since this type of medicinal has a great deal of qi and its flavor is penetrating and aromatic, they should not be boiled too long. Otherwise their medicinal effect will be decreased.

---

[1] I prefer to translate *ping* as level rather than Wiseman's calm since, I believe, the spatial dimension of the Chinese character is technically important to understanding this concept.

A. Acrid, warm exterior-resolving medicinals

Herba Ephedrae (*Ma Huang*)

Nature & flavor: Acrid, slightly bitter, and warm

Channel entry: Lungs and urinary bladder

Functions: Effuses sweat and resolves the exterior, diffuses the lungs and levels panting, disinhibits water and disperses swelling

Indications:

1. Used for external contraction of wind cold exterior conditions with symptoms of aversion to cold, fever (literally effusion or emission of heat), headache, nasal congestion, no sweating, and a floating, tight pulse. For this condition, Herba Ephedrae is commonly combined with Ramulus Cinnamomi Cassiae (*Gui Zhi*), Semen Pruni Armeniacae (*Xing Ren*), Radix Glycyrrhizae (*Gan Cao*). This is then called *Ma Huang Tang* (Ephedra Decoction).

2. Used for non-diffusion of the lung qi, coughing, panting, and rapid breathing. In this case, Herba Ephedrae is commonly combined with Semen Pruni Armeniacae (*Xing Ren*) and Radix Glycrrhizae (*Gan Cao*). This is then called *San Ao Tang* (Three Rough & Ready [Ingredients] Decoction). If there is cough and panting with profuse, thin, clear phlegm categorized as the lungs having cold rheum, then one can combine Herba Ephedrae with Herba Asari Cum Radice (*Xi Xin*), dry Rhizoma Zingiberis (*Gan Jiang*), Rhizoma Pinelliae Ternatae (*Ban Xia*), etc. as in *Xiao Qing Long Tang* (Minor Blue-green Dragon Decoction). If there is coughing and panting with fever categorized as heat evils blocking the lungs, then one can combine Herba Ephedrae with uncooked Gypsum Fibrosum (*Shi Gao*), Semen Pruni Armeniacae (*Xing Ren*), and Radix Glycyrrhizae (*Gan Cao*). This is called *Ma Xing Shi Gan Tang* (Ephedra, Armeniaca, Gypsum & Licorice Decoction).

3. Used for water swelling. If there is whole body edema and there is heat, one can combine Herba Ephedrae with uncooked Gypsum Fibrosum (*Shi Gao*) as in *Yue Bi Tang* (Effuse the Spleen Decoction). If there is water swelling, the pulse is deep, and there is cold, then one can combine Herba Ephedrae with Radix Lateralis Praeparatus Aconiti Carmichaeli (*Fu Zi*) and Radix Glycyrrhizae (*Gan Cao*). This is then called *Ma Huang Fu Zi Gan Cao Tang* (Ephedra, Aconite & Licorice Decoction).

Dosage: 1.5-10g

Method of use: Decoct in water and administer internally. For effusing sweat and

2

resolving the exterior, disinhibiting water and dispersing swelling, mostly use uncooked. For stopping cough and leveling panting, mostly use mix-fried.

Cautions & contraindications: This ingredient is a relatively strong sweat-effuser. Therefore, it is not appropriate to use in to large an amount. It is prohibited to use in exterior vacuity spontaneous perspiration, yin vacuity night sweats, and kidney not absorbing the qi vacuity panting. It should be used with care in those with insomnia and high blood pressure.

Ramulus Cinnamomi Cassiae (*Gui Zhi*)

Nature & flavor: Acrid, sweet, and warm

Channel entry: Lungs, heart, and urinary bladder

Functions: Effuses sweat and resolves the exterior, warms the channels and stops pain, invigorates yang and transforms the qi

Indications:

1. Used in external contraction wind cold with symptoms of headache, aversion to cold, etc. For exterior vacuity spontaneous perspiration, Ramulus Cinnamomi Cassiae is commonly combined with Radix Albus Paeoniae Lactiflorae (*Bai Shao*), uncooked Rhizoma Zingiberis (*Sheng Jiang*), Fructus Zizyphi Jujubae (*Da Zao*), and Radix Glycyrrhizae (*Gan Cao*). This is then called *Gui Zhi Tang* (Cinnamon Twig Decoction). For exterior repletion lack of sweating, one can combine Ramulus Cinnamomi Cassiae with Herba Ephedrae (*Ma Huang*), etc. as in *Ma Huang Tang* (Ephedra Decoction).

2. Used for wind cold damp impediment, shoulder, upper arm, and extremity joint soreness and pain. If wind dampness is in the exterior and exterior yang is tending to be vacuous, one can combine Ramulus Cinnamomi Cassiae with Radix Lateralis Praeparatus Aconiti Carmichaeli (*Fu Zi*), etc. as in *Gui Zhi Fu Zi Tang* (Cinnamon Twigs & Aconite Decoction). If there is an insufficiency of constructive and defensive qi with blood impediment stubborn numbness, one can combine Ramulus Cinnamomi Cassiae with Radix Astragali Membranacei (*Huang Qi*) and Radix Paeoniae Lactiflorae (*Shao Yao*) as in *Huang Qi Gui Zhi Wu Wu Tang* (Astragalus & Cinnamon Twig Five Materials Decoction).

3. Used for women's blood cold stasis and stagnation with menstrual irregularity, blocked menstruation, abdominal pain, and concretions and conglomerations, Ramulus Cinnamomi Cassiae is commonly combined with Radix Angelicae Sinensis (*Dang Gui*), Radix

Paeoniae (*Shao Yao*), Radix Ligustici Wallichii (*Chuan Xiong*), Semen Pruni Persicae (*Tao Ren*), Cortex Radicis Moutan (*Dan Pi*), and other such blood-quickening, freeing the flow of the channels medicinals as in *Wen Jing Tang* (Warm the Channels Decoction) or *Gui Zhi Fu Ling Wan* (Cinnamon Twigs & Poria Pills).

4. Used for middle burner vacuity cold with stomach and venter insidious pain with a liking for obtaining warmth and pressure. In that case, Ramulus Cinnamomi Cassiae is commonly combined with Radix Albus Paeoniae Lactiflorae (*Bai Shao*), Maltose (*Yi Tang*), and Radix Astragali Membranacei (*Huang Qi*) as in *Huang Qi Jian Zhong Tang* (Astragalus Fortify the Center Decoction).

5. Used for heart-spleen yang vacuity, yang qi not moving, with water dampness gathering internally. The symptoms of this are upper back pain and rib-side distention, cough counterflow, and dizziness. In that case, Ramulus Cinnamomi Cassiae is commonly combined with Sclerotium Poriae Cocos (*Fu Ling*) and Rhizoma Atractylodis Macrocephalae (*Bai Zhu*) as in *Ling Gui Zhu Gan Tang* (Poria, Cinnamon Twig, Atractylodes & Licorice Decoction). If there is urinary bladder qi transformation not moving inhibited urination and water swelling, Ramulus Cinnamomi Cassiae is commonly combined with Sclerotium Poriae Cocos (*Fu Ling*) and Sclerotium Polypori Umbellati (*Zhu Ling*) as in *Wu Ling San* (Five [Ingredients] Poria Powder).

6. Used for chest impediment and chest pain or heart stirring palpitations and a bound, regularly intermittent pulse. For the former, Ramulus Cinnamomi Cassiae is commonly combined with Fructus Immaturus Citri Aurantii (*Zhi Shi*), Fructus Trichosanthis Kirlowii (*Gua Lou*), and Bulbus Allii (*Xie Bai*) as in *Zhi Shi Xie Bai Gui Zhi Tang* (Immature Aurantium, Allium & Cinnamon Twig Decoction). For the latter, Ramulus Cinnamomi Cassiae is commonly combined with mix-fried Radix Glycyrrhizae (*Gan Cao*), Radix Panacis Ginseng (*Ren Shen*), and Gelatinum Corii Asini (*E Jiao*) as in *Zhi Gan Cao Tang* (Mix-fried Licorice Decoction).

Dosage: 3-10g

Method of use: Decoct in water and administer internally.

Cautions & contraindications: This ingredient is acrid and warm and it strengthens heat. Therefore, it easily damages yin and stirs the blood. This medicinal is contraindicated in warm heat diseases and yin vacuity-yang exuberance conditions, throat problems, or bleeding conditions or in those who habitually have fire internally with a dry mouth and tongue. It should be used cautiously in pregnant women and those with excessively profuse menstrual flow.

Herba Seu Flos Schizonepetae Tenuifoliae (*Jing Jie Sui*)

Nature & flavor: Acrid and slightly warm

Channel entry: Lungs and liver

Functions: Dispels wind and resolves the exterior, diffuses toxins and out-thrusts rashes, stops bleeding

Indications:

1. Used for external contraction wind cold with aversion to cold, fever, headache, no sweating, etc. In this case, Herba Seu Flos Schizonepetae Tenuifoliae is commonly combined with Radix Ledebouriellae Divaricatae (*Fang Feng*) and Radix Et Rhizoma Notopterygii (*Qiang Huo*) as in *Jing Fang Bai Du San* (Schizonepeta & Ledebouriella Vanquish Toxins Powder). It can also be used for the fever, headache, red eyes, and swollen throat of a wind heat exterior pattern. In that case, it is commonly combined with Flos Lonicerae Japonicae (*Jin Yin Hua*) Fructus Forsythiae Suspensae (*Lian Qiao*), Herba Menthae Haplocalycis (*Bo He*) and Radix Platycodi Grandiflori (*Jie Geng*) as in *Yin Qiao San* (Lonicera & Forsythia Powder).

2. Used for wind rashes and itching or measles rash which is not out-thrust easily or smoothly. For these purposes, Herba Seu Flos Schizonepetae Tenuifoliae is commonly combined with Herba Menthae Haplocalycis (*Bo He*), Periostracum Cicadae (*Chan Tui*), and Fructus Arctii Lappae (*Niu Bang Zi*). When used for the initial stage of sores and welling abscesses with an exterior pattern, it is commonly combined with Radix Ledebouriellae Divaricatae (*Fang Feng*), Flos Lonicerae Japonicae (*Jin Yin Hua*), Fructus Forsythiae Suspensae (*Lian Qiao*).

3. Used for spitting blood, spontaneous ejection of blood (*i.e.*, nosebleed), hemafecia, and flooding and leaking. In these cases, one can used carbonized Herba Seu Flos Schizonepetae Tenuifoliae combined with other stop-bleeding medicinals.

Dosage: 3-10g

Method of use: Decoct in water and administer internally. For effusing the exterior, one should use uncooked. For stopping bleeding, one should use stir-fried till carbonized.

Radix Ledebouriellae Divaricatae (*Fang Feng*)

Nature & flavor: Acrid and sweet, slightly warm

Channel entry: Urinary bladder, liver, and spleen

Functions: Scatters wind and resolves the exterior, overcomes dampness and stops pain, dispels wind and stops tetany

Indications:

1. Used for external contraction exterior conditions with headache and body pain. In those categorized as wind cold exterior patterns, Radix Ledebouriellae Divaricatae is commonly combined with Herba Seu Flos Schizonepetae Tenuifoliae (*Jing Jie Sui*). For those categorized as wind heat exterior patterns, it is commonly combined with Herba Menthae Haplocalycis (*Bo He*) and Fructus Forsythiae Suspensae (*Lian Qiao*). For those categorized as wind damp exterior patterns, it can be combined with Radix Et Rhizoma Notopterygii (*Qiang Huo*). If there is wind rash with itchy skin conditions, one can combine this medicinal with Herba Schizonepetae Tenuifoliae (*Jing Jie Sui*) and Fructus Tribuli Terrestris (*Bai Ji Li*).

2. Used for wind cold damp impediment, joint aching and pain, sinew vessel spasm and contraction. In that case, it is commonly combined with Radix Et Rhizoma Notopterygii (*Qiang Huo*) and Radix Angelicae Sinensis (*Dang Gui*) as in *Juan Bi Tang* (Alleviate Impediment Decoction).

3. Used for tetanus with arched back rigidity, clenched jaws, convulsions, and tetany. In that case, Radix Ledebouriellae Divaricatae is commonly combined with Rhizoma Arisaematis (*Tian Nan Xing*), Radix Aconiti Coreani Seu Typhonii (*Bai Fu Zi*), and Rhizoma Gastrodiae Elatae (*Tian Ma*) as in *Yu Zhen San* (Jade True Powder).

Dosage: 3-10g

Method of use: Decoct in water and administer internally.

Cautions & contraindications: This ingredient is mainly used for external wind. It should be used cautiously in blood vacuity stirring wind and yin vacuity fire effulgence.

Radix Et Rhizoma Notopterygii (*Qiang Huo*)

Nature & flavor: Acrid, bitter, and warm

Channel entry: Urinary bladder, liver, and kidneys

Functions: Resolves the exterior and scatters cold, dispels wind and overcomes dampness, stops pain

Indications:

1. Used for external contraction wind cold with aversion to cold, fever, headache, body pain, etc. In this case, Radix Et Rhizoma Notopterygii is commonly combined with Radix Ledebouriellae Divaricatae (*Fang Feng*), Radix Angelicae Dahuricae (*Bai Zhi*), and Herba Asari Cum Radice (*Xi Xin*) as in *Jiu Wei Qiang Huo Tang* (Nine Flavors Notopterygium Decoction).

2. Used for wind cold damp impediment with limb joint aching and pain. It is especially appropriate for aching and pain in the upper half of the body. In this case, Radix Et Rhizoma Notopeterygii is commonly combined with Radix Angelicae Pubescentis (*Du Huo*), Radix Ledebouriellae Divaricatae (*Fang Feng*), and Fructus Viticis (*Man Jing Zi*) as in *Qiang Huo Xing Shi Tang* (Notopterygium Overcome Dampness Decoction).

Dosage: 3-10g

Method of use: Decoct in water and administer internally.

Cautions & contraindications: This ingredient is upbearing, scattering, warming, and drying. Therefore, it easily damages yin and consumes the blood. It is contraindicated in those with qi and blood insufficiency patterns and those with external contractions with concomitant dry throats.

Radix Angelicae Dahuricae (*Bai Zhi*)

Nature & flavor: Acrid and warm

Channel entry: Lungs and stomach

Functions: Resolves the exterior and scatters cold, dispels wind and stops pain, disperses swelling and expels pus, transforms dampness and stops abnormal vaginal discharge

Indications:

1. Used for wind cold common cold with the symptoms of headache and nasal congestion. In this case, Radix Angelicae Dahuricae is commonly combined with Radix Ledebouriellae Divaricatae (*Fang Feng*) and Radix Et Rhizoma Notopterygii (*Qiang Huo*) as in *Jiu Wei Qiang Huo Tang* (Nine Flavors Notopterygium Decoction).

2. Used for headache and toothache. It is especially appropriate for forehead and superciliary bone pain. For the treatment of head wind and head pain, it is commonly combined with Radix Ligustici Wallichii (*Chuan Xiong*), Flos Chrysanthemi Morifolii (*Ju Hua*), and Radix Ledebouriellae Divaricatae (*Fang Feng*) as in *Chuan Xiong Cha Tiao San* (Ligusticum & Tea Mixed Powder). For the treatment of deep source nasal congestion and runny nose with pussy snivel and headache, it is commonly combined with Fructus Xanthii Sibirici (*Cang Er Zi*) and Flos Magnoliae Liliflorae (*Xin Yi*) as in *Cang Er Zi San* (Xanthium Powder). For the treatment of wind chill toothache where chill is heavy, one can combine Radix Angelicae Dahuricae with Herba Asari Cum Radice (*Xi Xin*). For wind heat toothache where heat is heavy, one can combine it with uncooked Gypsum Fibrosum (*Shi Gao*).

3. Used for sores and welling abscesses, swelling, and pain. For the treatment of breast abscess, Radix Angelicae Dahuricae is commonly combined with Fructus Trichosanthis Kirlowii (*Gua Lou*), Bulbus Fritillariae (*Bei Mu*), and Herba Taraxaci Mongolici Cum Radice (*Pu Gong Ying*). For the treatment of sores and swelling, it is commonly combined with Flos Lonicerae Japonicae (*Jin Yin Hua*) and Radix Trichosanthis Kirlowii (*Tian Hua Fen*).

4. Used for women's abnormal vaginal discharge conditions. For cold damp abnormal vaginal discharge which is profuse in amount and clear and thin in consistency, Radix Angelicae Dahuricae is commonly combined with Rhizoma Atractylodis Macrocephalae (*Bai Zhu*), Sclerotium Poriae Cocos (*Fu Ling*), and Os Sepiae Seu Sepiellae (*Hai Piao Xiao*). For damp heat abnormal vaginal discharge with foul odor, yellow color, and thick in consistency, one can combine it with Cortex Phellodendri (*Huang Bai*) and Semen Plantaginis (*Che Qian Zi*).

5. Used for stomach duct aching and pain. In this case, Radix Angelicae Dahuricae can be combined with Radix Glycyrrhizae (*Gan Cao*) as in *Bai Zhi Gan Cao Tang* (Angelica Dahurica & Licorice Decoction).

Dosage: 3-10g

Method of use: Decoct in water and administer internally.

Cautions & contraindications: When this medicinal is used in the treatment of stomach venter aching and pain, its amount can be as much as 30g. However, when the aching and pain are relaxed and resolved, its dosage should be decreased.

Folium Perillae Frutecentis (*Zi Su Ye*)

Nature & flavor: Acrid and warm

Channel entry: Lungs and spleen

Functions: Resolves the exterior and scatters cold, moves the qi and harmonizes the stomach

Indications:

1. Used for wind cold common cold with nasal congestion, cough, and profuse, white, watery phlegm, Folium Perillae Frutescentis is commonly combined with Radix Platycodi Grandiflori (*Jie Geng*) and Semen Prun Armeniacae (*Xing Ren*).

2. Used for dampness and phlegm obstructing the middle burner vomiting and nausea, Folium Perillae Frutescentis is commonly combined with Fructus Amomi (*Sha Ren*) especially in the treatment of nausea and vomiting during pregnancy.

3. Used for seafood poisoning, this medicinal is often combined with uncooked Rhizoma Zingiberis (*Sheng Jiang*).

Dosage: 6-12g

Method of use: Decoct in water and administer internally.

Cautions & contraindications: This medicinal is not appropriate for use in exterior vacuity conditions with profuse sweating.

Radix Et Rhizoma Ligustici Chinensis (*Gao Ben*)

Nature & flavor: Acrid and warm

Channel entry: Urinary bladder

Functions: Dispels wind and scatters cold, eliminates dampness and stops pain

Indications: Used for wind cold headache with pain at the vertex, stiff neck, or toothache, Radix Et Rhizoma Ligustici Chinensis is commonly combined with Herba Asari Cum Radice (*Xi Xin*). If pain and stiffness are due to wind, cold, and dampness, this medicinal can be combined with Rhizoma Atractylodis (*Cang Zhu*).

Dosage: 3-10g

Method of use: Decoct in water and administer internally.

Cautions & contraindications: Due to its relatively strong drying nature, this medicinal is not appropriate for use in cases of yin and blood vacuity.

Herba Asari Cum Radice (*Xi Xin*)

Nature & flavor: Acrid and warm

Channel entry: Lungs, spleen, and kidneys

Functions: Dispels wind and scatters cold, frees the flow of the network vessels and stops pain, warms the lungs and transforms rheum

Indications:

1. Used for wind cold conditions with coughing and panting and profuse phlegm, Herba Asari Cum Radice can be combined with Herba Ephedrae (*Ma Huang*).

2. Used for wind cold external contraction headache, Herba Asari Cum Radice can be combined with Radix Bupleuri (*Chai Hu*).

3. Used for wind heat headache and toothache, Herba Asari Cum Radice is often combined with uncooked Radix Rehmanniae (*Sheng Di*).

4. Used for chest pain and breast nodes. For the former, Herba Asari Cum Radice is commonly combined with Ramulus Cinnamomi Cassiae (*Gui Zhi*) and Radix Salviae Miltiorrhizae (*Dan Shen*). For the latter, it is commonly combined with Radix Angelicae Sinensis (*Dang Gui*) and Flos Carthami Tinctorii (*Hong Hua*).

In addition, this medicinal can also be used externally for the treatment of sores arising within the mouth.

Dosage: 1-3g. Externally, use a suitable amount.

Method of use: Decoct in water and administer internally. For sores in the mouth, grind into fine powder, mix with water, and apply to the affected area, or mix with a decoction of Rhizoma Coptidis Chinensis (*Huang Lian*) and apply externally.

Uncooked Rhizoma Zingiberis (*Sheng Jiang*)

Nature & flavor: Acrid and slightly warm

Channel entry: Lungs, spleen, and stomach

Functions: Resolves the exterior and scatters cold, warms the center and stops vomiting, transforms phlegm and stops cough

Indications:

1. Used for wind cold external contraction with coughing and panting, runny nose, and nasal congestion, uncooked Rhizoma Zingiberis is commonly combined with Herba Ephedrae (*Ma Huang*) as in *Ma Huang Tang* (Ephedra Decoction).

2. Used for damp phlegm obstructing the center resulting in stomach duct and abdominal fullness and oppression and nausea and vomiting, uncooked Rhizoma Zingiberis is commonly combined with Rhizoma Pinelliae Ternatae (*Ban Xia*) and Sclerotium Poriae Cocos (*Fu Ling*) as in *Er Chen Tang* (Two Aged [Ingredients] Decoction). If there is accompanying heat in the stomach, it may be combined with Rhizoma Coptidis Chinensis (*Huang Lian*) and Radix Scutellariae Baicalensis (*Huang Qin*) as in *Sheng Jiang Xie Xin Tang* (Uncooked Ginger Drain the Heart Decoction).

Dosage: 3-10g

Method of use: Decoct in water and administer internally, added later. It may also be rubbed on the tongue as a first aid treatment for nausea.

Note: Uncooked Succus Zingiberis (*Sheng Jiang Zhi*)'s acrid scattering power is stronger. Its function is to open phlegm and stop vomiting. It is mostly used for wind stroke phlegm confounding with locked jaws and clouding reversal or for incessant vomiting. For these purposes, 3-10 drops are mixed in with decoctions. Uncooked Cortex Rhizomatis Zingiberis (*Sheng Jiang Pi*) is acrid and cool. Its functions are to move water. It mainly treats skin water swelling. It is used in doses of 3-6g. Roasted Rhizoma Zingiberis (*Wei Jiang*)'s acrid scattering is not as extreme as uncooked Ginger's. It is better than uncooked Ginger for warming the center and stopping vomiting and is suitable for spleen-stomach vacuity cold abdominal pain and vomiting or diarrhea. It is used in doses of 3-10g.

Flos Magnoliae Liliflorae (*Xin Yi Hua*)

Nature & flavor: Acrid and warm

Channel entry: Lungs

Functions: Scatters wind cold and frees the flow of the portals of the nose

Indications: Used for nasal congestion, runny nose, and deep source nasal congestion. For conditions categorized as wind cold, Flos Magnoliae Liliflorae is commonly combined with Fructus Xanthii Sibirici (*Cang Er Zi*), Radix Angelicae Dahuricae (*Bai Zhi*), and Herba Asari Cum Radice (*Xi Xin*). For heat conditions, it can be combined with Gypsum Fibrosum (*Shi Gao*), Radix Scutellariae Baicalensis (*Huang Qin*), and Herba Menthae Haplocalycis (*Bo He*). For pain above and around the eyes categorized as wind heat, this medicinal can be combined with Flos Chrysanthemi Morifolii (*Ju Hua*) and Herba Siegesbeckiae (*Xi Xian Cao*).

Dosage: 3-10g

Method of use: Decoct in water and administer internally.

B. Acrid, cool exterior-resolving medicinals

Herba Menthae Haplocalycis (*Bo He*)

Nature & flavor: Acrid and cool

Channel entry: Lungs and liver

Functions: Courses and scatters wind heat, clears the head and eyes, disinhibits the throat, out-thrusts rashes and stops itching

Indications:

1. Used for external contraction wind heat and the initial stage of warm diseases. The symptoms manifest in that case are slight aversion to cold, headache, no sweating, etc. Thus Herba Menthae Haplocalycis is commonly combined with Flos Lonicerae Japonicae (*Yin Hua*) and Fructus Forsythiae Suspensae (*Lian Qiao*) as in *Yin Qiao San* (Lonicera & Forsythia Powder). If there is a summertime affection of summerheat heat with fever, dizziness, oral thirst, and short, reddish urination, one can combine Herba Menthae

Haplocalycis with Talcum (*Hua Shi*) and Radix Glycyrrhizae (*Gan Cao*) as in *Ji Su San* (Peppermint Powder).

2. Used for wind heat common cold or wind fire attacking above leading to the arising of headache, red eyes, and a swollen, painful throat. In that case, Herba Menthae Haplocalycis is commonly combined with Flos Chrysanthemi Morifolii (*Ju Hua*), Fructus Arctii Lappae (*Niu Bang Zi*), Radix Platycodi Grandiflori (*Jie Geng*), and Herba Seu Flos Schizonepetae Tenuifoliae (*Jing Jie Sui*).

3. Used for the initial stage of measles, wind heat externally lodged in the muscles and exterior with a rash that is not easily or smoothly out-thrust, or wind rash with itchy skin, etc. In that case, this medicinal is commonly combined with Fructus Forsythiae Suspensae (*Lian Qiao*), Periostacum Cicadae (*Chan Tui*), and Fructus Arctii Lappae (*Niu Bang Zi*).

In addition, this medicinal can be combined with Radix Albus Paeoniae Lactiflorae (*Bai Shao*) and Radix Bupleuri (*Chai Hu*) for the treatment of liver qi depression and stagnation with chest oppression and rib-side and flank distention and pain as in *Xiao Yao San* (Rambling Powder).

Dosage: 3-10g. Fresh, this medicinal can be used in doses of 15-30g.

Method of use: Decoct in water and administer internally, adding later. For effusing and scattering wind heat, mostly use the leaves. For rectifying the qi and soothing the liver, mostly use the stems.

Cautions & contraindications: This medicinal should not be used if there is exterior vacuity spontaneous perspiration.

Folium Mori Albi (*Sang Ye*)

Nature & flavor: Sweet, bitter, and cold

Channel entry: Lungs and liver

Functions: Courses and scatters wind heat, clears the lungs and stops cough, clears the liver and brightens the eyes

Indications:

1. Used for external contraction of wind heat or the initial stage of a warm disease with the symptoms of fever, dizziness, headache, cough, and a swollen, painful throat. In this case,

Folium Mori Albi is commonly combined with Flos Chrysanthemi Morifolii (*Ju Hua*), Fructus Forsythiae Suspensae (*Lian Qiao*), and Radix Platycodi Grandiflori (*Jie Geng*) as in *Sang Ju Yin* (Morus & Chrysanthemum Drink).

2. Used for dry heat damaging the lungs with the symptoms of cough, thick phlegm, and dryness of the nose and throat. In this case, Folium Mori Albi is commonly combined with Semen Pruni Armeniacae (*Xing Ren*), Bulbus Fritillariae (*Bei Mu*), and Tuber Ophiopogonis Japonici (*Mai Men Dong*) as in *Sang Xing Tang* (Morus & Armeniaca Decoction) and *Qing Zao Jiu Fei Tang* (Clear Dryness & Rescue the Lungs Decoction).

3. Used for liver channel replete heat or wind heat causing red, rough, dry eyes and profuse tearing. In that case, Folium Mori Albi is commonly combined with Flos Chrysanthemi Morifolii (*Ju Hua*) and Semen Cassiae Torae (*Jue Ming Zi*). If categorized as liver yin insufficiency with dimness, clouding, and blurring of vision, one can combine this medicinal with black Semen Sesami Indici (*Hei Zhi Ma*) processed into honey pills and administered over an enduring period of time, such as in *Sang Ma Wan* (Morus & Sesame Pills).

Dosage: 6-12g

Method of use: Decoct in water and administer internally or take as pills or powder.

Flos Chrysanthemi Morifolii (*Ju Hua*)

Nature & flavor: Sweet, slightly bitter, and slightly cold

Channel entry: Liver and lungs

Functions: Courses wind and clears heat, levels the liver and brightens the eyes

Indications:

1. Used for external contraction wind heat and the initial stage of warm diseases. The symptoms of this are fever, dizziness, and headache. In that case, Flos Chrysanthemi Morifolii is commonly combined with Folium Mori Albi (*Sang Ye*), Herba Menthae Haplocalycis (*Bo He*), and Fructus Forsythiae Suspensae (*Lian Qiao*) as in *Sang Ju Yin* (Morus & Chrysanthemum Drink).

2. Used for liver channel wind heat or liver fire attacking upward resulting in red, swollen, painful eyes. In that case, this medicinal is commonly combined with Folium Mori Albi (*Sang Ye*), Periostracum Cicadae (*Chan Tui*), and Spica Prunellae Vulgaris (*Xia Ku Cao*).

14

3. Used for ascendant liver yang hyperactivity manifest as headache, dizziness, and distention of the head. In that case, Flos Chrysanthemi Morifolii is commonly combined with Cornu Caprae (*Shan Yang Jiao*), Ramulus Uncariae Cum Uncis (*Gou Teng*), and uncooked Radix Rehmanniae (*Sheng Di*) as in *Ling Jiao Gou Teng Tang* (Antelope Horn & Uncaria Decoction).[2] If there is liver-kidney yin vacuity with clouded, blurred vision, then this medicinal is commonly combined with cooked Radix Rehmanniae (*Shu Di*) and Fructus Lycii Chinensis (*Gou Qi Zi*) as in *Qi Ju Di Huang Wan* (Lycium & Chrysanthemum Rehmannia Pills).

Dosage: 10-15g

Method of use: Steep in boiling water or take as powder or pills. For coursing wind and clearing heat, mostly use yellow Flos Chrysanthemi Morifolii (*Huang Ju Hua*), while for leveling the liver and brightening the eyes, mostly use white Flos Chrysanthemi Morifolii (*Bai Ju Hua*).

Radix Puerariae (*Ge Gen*)

Nature & flavor: Sweet, acrid, and cool

Channel entry: Spleen and stomach

Functions: Resolves the muscles and recedes or abates heat, engenders fluids and stops thirst, out-thrusts and effuses measles rash, upbears yang and stops diarrhea

Indications:

1. Used for external contraction exterior patterns whose symptoms are fever, headache, no sweating, neck and upper back stiffness and pain. For wind cold exterior patterns, Radix Puerariae is commonly combined with Herba Ephedrae (*Ma Huang*), Ramulus Cinnamomi Cassiae (*Gui Zhi*), and Radix Albus Paeoniae Lactiflorae (*Bai Shao*) as in *Ge Gen Tang* (Pueraria Decoction). For wind heat exterior patterns with simultaneous internal heat, Radix Puerariae can be combined with Radix Scutellariae Baicalensis (*Huang Qin*), Gypsum Fibrosum (*Shi Gao*), and Radix Bupleuri (*Chai Hu*) as in *Chai Ge Jie Ji Tang* (Bupleurum & Pueraria Resolves the Muscles Decoction).

2. Used for heat disease vexatious thirst and wasting thirst condition with oral dryness and profuse drinking. In that case, Radix Puerariae may be used alone or combined with Tuber

---

[2] Historically, this formula's main ingredient was Cornu Antelopis Saiga-tatarici (*Ling Yang Jiao*). However, because this ingredient comes from an endangered species, it should always be substituted with goat horn.

Ophiopogonis Japonici (*Mai Men Dong*), Radix Trichosanthis Kirlowii (*Tian Hua Fen*), and Radix Rehmanniae (*Di Huang*) as in *Yu Quan San* (Jade Spring Powder).

3. Used for the initial stage of measles with fever, aversion to cold, and uneasy or unsmoothly exiting of the rash. In that case, Radix Puerariae is commonly combined with Rhizoma Cimicifugae (*Sheng Ma*) and Radix Paeoniae Lactiflorae (*Shao Yao*) as in *Sheng Ma Ge Gen Tang* (Cimicifuga & Pueraria Decoction).

4. Used for damp heat diarrhea and dysentery or spleen vacuity diarrhea. In the former case, Radix Pueraria is commonly combined with Radix Scutellariae Baicalensis (*Huang Qin*) and Rhizoma Coptidis Chinensis (*Huang Lian*) as in *Ge Gen Qin Lian Tang* (Pueraria, Scutellaria & Coptis Decoction). In the latter case, it is commonly combined with Radix Panacis Ginseng (*Ren Shen*), Rhizoma Atractylodis Macrocephalae (*Bai Zhu*), and Radix Auklandiae Lappae (*Mu Xiang*) as in *Qi Wei Bai Zhu San* (Seven Flavors Atractylodes Powder).

In addition, this medicinal has recently been used for hypertensive cerebral disease with the symptoms of headache, dizziness, and stiff neck with some effect.

Dosage: 10-20g

Method of use: Decoct in water and administer internally or take as pills or powder. For stopping diarrhea, one should use roasted. Otherwise, one should use uncooked.

Radix Bupleuri (*Chai Hu*)

Nature & flavor: Bitter, acrid, and slightly cold

Channel entry: Liver and gallbladder

Functions: Out-thrusts the exterior and recedes or abates heat, courses the liver and resolves depression, upbears and lifts the yang qi

Indications:

1. Used for common cold fever and damage due to cold evils located in the *shao yang* with alternating cold and heat (*i.e.*, fever and chills), chest and rib-side bitterness and fullness, a bitter taste in the mouth, and dry throat. In the first case, Radix Bupleuri is commonly used with Radix Glycyrrhizae (*Gan Cao*) as in *Chai Hu San* (Bupleurum Powder) or with Radix Puerariae (*Ge Gen*) as in *Chai Ge Jie Ji Tang* (Bupleurum & Pueraria Resolve the Muscles Decoction). In the latter case, it is combined with Radix Scutellariae Baicalensis

(*Huang Qin*), Rhizoma Pinelliae Ternatae (*Ban Xia*), and Radix Codonopsitis Pilosulae (*Dang Shen*) as in *Xiao Chai Hu Tang* (Minor Bupleurum Decoction).

2. Used for liver depression qi stagnation, the symptoms of which are chest and diaphragmatic fullness and oppression, rib-side and flank distention and pain. In that case, Radix Bupleuri is commonly combined with Rhizoma Cyperi Rotundi (*Xiang Fu*), Radix Ligustici Wallichii (*Chuan Xiong*), and Fructus Citri Aurantii (*Zhi Ke*) as in *Chai Hu Shu Gan San* (Bupleurum Course the Liver Powder). If there is liver depression blood vacuity with menstrual irregularities, one can combine Radix Bupleuri with Radix Angelicae Sinensis (*Dang Gui*) and Radix Albus Paeoniae Lactiflorae (*Bai Shao*) as in *Xiao Yao San* (Rambling Powder).

3. Used for qi vacuity downward fall resulting in anal prolapse, uterine prolapse, and stomach ptosis or shortness of qi exhaustion and fatigue. In that case, Radix Bupleuri is commonly combined with Radix Panacis Ginseng (*Ren Shen*), Radix Astragali Membranacei (*Huang Qi*), and Rhizoma Cimicifugae (*Sheng Ma*) as in *Bu Zhong Yi Qi Tang* (Supplement the Center & Boost the Qi Decoction).

In addition, when this ingredient is combined with Radix Scutellariae Baicalensis (*Huang Qin*) and Radix Dichroae Febrifugae (*Chang Shan*), it is effective for the treatment of malaria.

Dosage: 3-10g. In order to recede fever, one can use this ingredient at doses of 15-30g.

Method of use: Decoct in water and administer internally. Stir-frying this medicinal in vinegar is able to reduce its scattering nature and increase its action of stopping pain.

Cautions & contraindications: This ingredient's nature and action is upbearing and effusing. Therefore, it is contraindicated in yin vacuity fire effulgence and ascendant hyperactivity of liver yang tinnitus, deafness, dizziness, and headache.

Fructus Arctii Lappae (*Niu Bang Zi*)

Nature & flavor: Acrid, bitter, and cold

Channel entry: Lungs and stomach

Functions: Courses and scatters wind heat, diffuses the lungs and out-thrusts rashes, resolves toxins and disinhibits the throat

Indications:

1. Used for wind heat external contraction sore, swollen throat, and hoarse voice, Fructus Arctii Lappae is commonly combined with Radix Platycodi Grandiflori (*Jie Geng*) and Herba Menthae Haplocalycis (*Bo He*).

2. Used for the initial stage of sores with swelling and pain which have not yet ulcerated, Fructus Arctii Lappae can be combined with Radix Angelicae Dahuricae (*Bai Zhi*), Radix Platycodi Grandiflori (*Jie Geng*), and Flos Lonicerae Japonicae (*Jin Yin Hua*).

3. Used for measles rash which is not out-thrust smoothly or easily or for urticaria, Fructus Arctii Lappae can be combined with Herba Seu Flos Schizonepetae Tenuifoliae (*Jing Jie*), Radix Ledebouriellae Divaricatae (*Fang Feng*), and Flos Lonicerae Japonicae (*Jin Yin Hua*).

Dosage: 6-12g

Method of use: Decoct in water and administer internally.

Cautions & contraindications: Because this medicinal has the effect of clearing the intestines and freeing the flow of the stool, it should be used cautiously in case of loose stools.

Periostracum Cicadae (*Chan Tui*)

Nature & flavor: Sweet, salty, and cold

Channel entry: Lungs and liver

Functions: Scatters wind and eliminates heat, disinhibits the throat, out-thrusts rashes, recedes eye screen, and resolves tetany

Indications:

1. Used for the initial stage of wind heat rashes with itching, Periostracum Cicadae is commonly combined with Herba Menthae Haplocalycis (*Bo He*).

2. Used for red, itchy eyes or corneal opacity, Periostracum Cicadae may be combined with Flos Chrysanthemi Morifolii (*Ju Hua*) and Folium Mori Albi (*Sang Ye*).

3. Used for lung heat sore throat, Periostracum Cicadae can be combined with Semen Sterculiae Scaphageriae (*Pang Da Hai*).

4. Used for tetanus with locked jaws, and arched back rigidity, Periostracum Cicadae is commonly combined with Rhizoma Gastrodiae Elatae (*Tian Ma*) and Buthus Martensis (*Quan Xie*). For children's fright wind and febrile convulsions, it is commonly combined with Ramulus Uncariae Cum Uncis (*Gou Teng*), Radix Scutellariae Baicalensis (*Huang Qin*), and Cornu Caprae (*Shan Yang Jiao*).[3]

Dosage: 3-10g. For dispelling wind and resolving tetany, this medicinal may be used in doses of 15-30g.

Method of use: Decoct in water and administer internally.

Cautions & contraindications: This medicinal is not appropriate for use in exterior vacuity conditions. It should be used cautiously in pregnant women.

Fructus Viticis (*Man Jing Zi*)

Nature & flavor: Bitter, acrid, and slightly cold

Channel entry: Liver, stomach, and urinary bladder

Functions: Courses and scatters wind heat, clears and disinhibits the vertex and eyes

Indications:

1. Used for wind heat resulting in headache and eye pain, Fructus Viticis is commonly combined with Flos Chrysanthemi Morifolii (*Ju Hua*).

2. Used for external contraction of wind dampness resulting in headache, upper back, and back of the neck pain, Fructus Viticis is commonly combined with Radix Ligustici Wallichii (*Chuan Xiong*) and Radix Ledebouriellae Divaricatae (*Fang Feng*).

Dosage: 6-12g

Method of use: Decoct in water and administer internally

Cautions & contraindications: Use cautiously for headache and eye diseases due to yin or blood vacuity. Use cautiously in those with stomach qi vacuity.

---

[3]Traditionally, this combination uses Cornu Antelopis Saiga-tatarici (*Ling Yang Jiao*). However, this is an endangered species and can easily and effectively be substituted with goat horn.

Semen Praeparatum Sojae (*Dan Dou Chi*)

Nature & flavor: Acrid, sweet, and cool

Channel entry: Lungs and stomach

Functions: Resolves the exterior, eliminates vexation, and recedes fever or abates heat

Indications:

1. Used for the initial stage of wind heat conditions with fever, slight aversion to wind, sweating, and sore, swollen throat, Semen Praeparatum Sojae is commonly combined with Flos Lonicerae Japonicae (*Jin Yin Hua*), Fructus Forsythiae Suspensae (*Lian Qiao*), and Herba Menthae Haplocalycis (*Bo He*).

2. Used for the latter stage of heat disease with heat damaging yin fluids resulting in vexation and insomnia, Semen Praeparatum Sojae is often combined with Fructus Gardeniae Jasminoidis (*Zhi Zi*).

Dosage: 10-15g

Method of use: Decoct in water and administer internally.

Herba Equiseti Hiemalis (*Mu Zei*)

Nature & flavor: Sweet, bitter, and level

Channel entry: Lungs and liver

Functions: Scatters wind heat and recedes eye screen

Indications: Used for redness, swelling, and pain of the eyes, Herba Equiseti Hiemalis, can be combined with Flos Chrysanthemi Morifolii (*Ju Hua*). For itching of the eyes and profuse tearing, it may be combined with Fructus Tribuli Terrestris (*Bai Ji Li*). For blurred vision and profuse tearing, it may be combined with Rhizoma Atractylodis (*Cang Zhu*).

Dosage: 3-10g

Method of use: Decoct in water and administer internally.

Cautions & contraindications: Use cautiously in those with frequent urination, fluid consumption, or qi vacuity. Use cautiously in pregnant women.

Rhizoma Cimicifugae (*Sheng Ma*)

Nature & flavor: Acrid, slightly sweet, and slightly cold

Channel entry: Lungs, spleen, stomach, and large intestine

Functions: Effuses the exterior and out-thrusts rashes, clears heat and resolves toxins, upbears and lifts yang qi

Indications:

1. Used for the emission stage of measles when the rash is emitting uneasily or unsmoothly, Rhizoma Cimicifugae is commonly combined with Radix Puerariae (*Ge Gen*) as in *Sheng Ma Ge Gen Tang* (Cimicifuga & Pueraria Decoction).

2. Used for central qi downward fall resulting in stomach prolapse, anal prolapse, enduring hemorrhoids, uterine prolapse, abnormal vaginal discharge, flooding and leaking ,and enduring diarrhea and dysentery, Rhizoma Cimicifugae is commonly combined with Radix Bupleuri (*Chai Hu*) as in *Bu Zhong Yi Qi Tang* (Supplement the Center & Boost the Qi Decoction).

3. Used for heart-spleen fire resulting in the arising of sores on the tongue and within the mouth, Rhizoma Cimicifugae is often combined with Rhizoma Coptidis Chinensis (*Huang Lian*).

Dosage: 3-10g

Method of use: Decoct in water and administer internally. For resolving the exterior, use uncooked. For lifting fallen central qi, use mix-fried.

2

Heat-clearing medicinals

Medicinals whose main action is to clear and discharge internal heat are called heat-clearing medicinals. The natures of all heat-clearing medicinals are either cold or cool. They are mainly suitable for use in heat disease high fever, heat dysentery, welling abscess swelling, sores, and toxins, and yin vacuity internal heat types of interior heat patterns.

Heat-clearing medicinals can be categorized into six different types: those which clear heat and discharge fire, those which clear heat and dry dampness, those which clear heat and cool the blood, those which clear heat and resolve toxins, those which clear and abate or recede vacuity heat, and those which clear heat and resolve summerheat. Thus, for different types of internal heat, different types of heat-clearing medicinals should be chosen.

Because heat-clearing medicinals are cold or cool in nature, they easily damage yang and vanquish the stomach. Therefore, if yang qi is insufficient or there is spleen-stomach vacuity cold, or poor stomach grasping or absorption, heat-clearing medicinals should be used cautiously. In addition, the use of heat-clearing medicinals should be stopped as soon as possible so as to prevent damaging and causing detriment to the righteous qi.

A. Heat-clearing, fire-draining medicinals

Heat-clearing, fire draining medicinals mainly clear fire and heat from the qi division. They are suitable for use for strong heat or fever, sweating, oral thirst, vexation and agitation, delirious speech, mania, short, reddish urination, dry, yellow tongue fur, and a surging, replete, forceful pulse showing an interior heat blazing and exuberant pattern.

Gypsum Fibrosum (*Shi Gao*)

Nature & flavor: Acrid, sweet, and greatly cold

Channel entry: Lungs and stomach

Functions: Clears heat and drains fire, eliminates vexation and stops thirst, engenders muscles and restrains sores

Indications:

1. Used for acute heat diseases with evils located in the qi division, the symptoms of which manifest as strong heat (or fever), vexation and agitation, oral thirst with a desire to drink, perspiration, a surging, large pulse and other such symptoms of replete heat effulgence and exuberance. In this case, Gypsum Fibrosum is commonly combined with Rhizoma Anemarrhenae Aspheloidis (*Zhi Mu*), Semen Oryzae Sativae (*Geng Mi*), and Radix Glycyrrhizae (*Gan Cao*) as in *Bai Hu Tang* (White Tiger Decoction). If heat toxins are blocking and exuberant with a high fever which does not recede and the emission of macules and rashes, one can combine this medicinal with Cornu Bubali (*Shui Niu Jiao*) and Radix Scrophulariae Ningpoensis (*Xuan Shen*) as in *Hua Ban Tang* (Transform Macules Decoction). In the later stage of a warm disease with remaining heat which has not been cleared and the symptoms of heart vexation, dry mouth, and a red tongue with scanty fur, one can combine Gypsum Fibrosum with Folium Bambusae (*Zhu Ye*) and Tuber Ophiopogonis Japonici (*Mai Men Dong*) as in *Zhu Ye Shi Gao Tang* (Bamboo Leaf & Gypsum Decoction).

2. Used for lung heat repletion panting with distressed, rapid respiration, heart vexation, and oral thirst, Gypsum Fibrosum is commonly combined with Herba Ephedrae (*Ma Huang*), Semen Pruni Armeniacae (*Xing Ren*), and Radix Glycyrrhizae (*Gan Cao*) as in *Ma Xing Shi Gan Tang* (Ephedra, Armeniaca, Gypsum & Licorice Decoction).

3. Used for stomach fire flaring upward resulting in headache and swelling and pain of the gums of the teeth, Gypsum Fibrosum is commonly combined with uncooked Radix Rehmanniae (*Sheng Di*), Radix Achyranthis Bidentatae (*Niu Xi*), and Rhizoma Anemarrhenae Aspheloidis (*Zhi Mu*) as in *Yu Nu Jian* (Jade Women Decoction).

4. When used for sores and open sores weeping and not being constrained *i.e.*, not pulling together to heal, eczema, burns and scalds, Gypsum is fire calcined, ground into powder, and used externally. It then treats mouth sores not restrained and difficulty engendering new flesh. In that case, it is commonly combined with upbearing medicinals such as in *Jiu Yi Dan* (Nine [to] One Elixir).

Dosage: 15-60g. In larger doses, this ingredient may be used up to 120g. Externally, use a suitable amount.

Method of use: Decoct in water and administer internally. One should decoct it first. To clear heat and drain fire, one should use uncooked, while to engender flesh and restrain sores, one should use calcined.

Cautions & contraindications: This medicinal is contraindicated in spleen-stomach vacuity cold and yin vacuity internal heat.

Rhizoma Anemarrhenae Aspheloidis (*Zhi Mu*)

Nature & flavor: Bitter, sweet, and cold

Channel entry: Lungs, stomach, and kidneys

Functions: Clears heat and drains fire, enriches yin and moistens dryness, engenders fluids and stops thirst

Indications:

1. Used for warm heat disease whose symptoms are high fever, vexatious thirst, and a surging, large pulse, Rhizoma Anemarrhenae Aspheloidis is commonly combined with Gypsum Fibrosum (*Shi Gao*) as in *Bai Hu Tang* (White Tiger Decoction).

2. Used for lung heat cough or yin vacuity dry cough with thick phlegm, Rhizoma Anemarrhenae Aspheloidis is commonly combined with Bulbus Fritillariae (*Bei Mu*) as in *Er Mu San* (Two Mu's Powder).

3. Used for yin vacuity fire effulgence with symptoms of bone steaming and tidal heat, heart vexation, and night sweats, Rhizoma Anemarrhenae Aspheloidis is commonly combined with Cortex Phellodendri (*Huang Bai*) and uncooked Radix Rehmanniae (*Sheng Di*) as in *Zhi Bai Di Huang Wan* (Anemarrhena & Phellodendron Rehmannia Pills).

4. Used for yin vacuity wasting and thirsting with the symptoms of oral thirst, polydipsia, and polyuria, This medicinal is commonly combined with Radix Trichosanthis Kirlowii (*Tian Hua Fen*), Tuber Ophiopogonis Japonici (*Mai Men Dong*), and Radix Puerariae (*Ge Gen*) as in *Yu Ye Tang* (Jade Humor Decoction).

Dosage: 3-12g

Method of use: Decoct in water and administer internally. Mostly this ingredient is used uncooked. When it is stir-fried and processed in salt water, it enters the kidneys and drains fire.

Cautions & contraindications: This ingredient's nature is cold and its substance is moist. It is able to make slippery the intestines. Therefore, it is not appropriate to use it with spleen vacuity loose stools.

Fructus Gardeniae Jasminoidis (*Zhi Zi*)

Nature & flavor: Bitter and cold

Channel entry: Heart, lungs, stomach, and triple burner

Functions: Drains fire and eliminates vexation, clears heat and disinhibits dampness, cools the blood and stops bleeding

Indications:

1. Used for heat disease heart vexation, depression and oppression, agitation and restlessness, this medicinal is commonly combined with Semen Praeparatus Sojae (*Dan Dou Chi*) which is then called *Zhi Zi Chi Tang* (Gardenia & Soya Decoction). If heat toxins have accumulated and are exuberant with symptoms of high fever, vexation and agitation, spirit clouding, and delirious speech, this medicinal is commonly combined with Rhizoma Coptidis Chinensis (*Huang Lian*) and Radix Scutellariae Baicalensis (*Huang Qin*) as in *Qing Wen Bai Du Yin* (Clear the Scourge & Vanquish Toxins Drink).

2. Used for liver-gallbladder damp heat depression and binding with fever, jaundice, and short, reddish urination, Fructus Gardeniae Jasminoidis is commonly combined with Herba Artemisiae Capillaris (*Yin Chen Hao*), Radix Et Rhizoma Rhei (*Da Huang*), and Cortex Phellodendri (*Huang Bai*) as in *Yin Chen Hao Tang* (Capillaris Decoction) and *Zhi Zi Bai Pi Tang* (Gardenia & Phellodendron Decoction).

3. Used for blood heat frenetically moving spitting of blood, spontaneous ejection of blood, precipitation of blood with dysentry, or hematuria, Fructus Gardeniae Jasminoidis (*Zhi Zi*) is commonly combined with Rhizoma Imperatae Cylindricae (*Bai Mao Gen*), uncooked Radix Rehmanniae (*Sheng Di*), and Radix Scutellariae Baicalensis (*Huang Qin*).

In addition, uncooked Fructus Gardeniae Jasminoidis can be ground into powder, mixed with vinegar, and applied externally for the treatment of injury due to fall and strike with blood stasis, swelling, and pain. If ground into powder and mixed with egg whites, it can be applied externally to treat scalds and burns.

Dosage: 3-10g. Externally, use a suitable amount.

Method of use: Decoct in water and administer internally. For clearing heat and draining fire, one should use uncooked. For cooling the blood and stopping bleeding, one should use stir-fried till carbonized. For stopping vexation and vomiting, use stir-fried with ginger juice.

Herba Lophatheri Gracilis (*Dan Zhu Ye*)[4]

Nature & flavor: Sweet, bland, and cold

Channel entry: Heart, stomach, and urinary bladder

Functions: Clears heat and eliminates vexation, disinhibits urination

Indications:

1. Used for late stage heat diseases with a fever which will not abate, vexatious heat, a desire for chilled drinks, and a red tongue with scanty fur, Herba Lophatheri Gracilis is commonly combined with Gypsum Fibrosum (*Shi Gao*) as in *Zhu Ye Shi Gao Tang* (Bamboo Leaf & Gypsum Decoction).

2. Used for heat in the heart channel resulting in vexation, sores in the mouth and on the tongue, and reddish, scanty urination, Herba Lophatheri Gracilis can be combined with Caulis Akebiae (*Mu Tong*) and uncooked Radix Rehmanniae (*Sheng Di*) as in *Dao Chi San* (Abduct the Red Powder).

Dosage: 6-12g

Method of use: Decoct in water and administer internally.

Spica Prunellae Vulgaris (*Xia Ku Cao*)

Nature & flavor: Bitter, acrid, and cold

Channel entry: Liver, gallbladder, and lungs

Functions: Clears fire, brightens the eyes, scatters nodulations, and disperses swelling

Indications:

1. Used for redness, swelling, and pain in the eyes, Spica Prunellae Vulgaris is commonly combined with Flos Chrysanthemi Morifolii (*Ju Hua*).

2. Used for scrofulous phlegm kernels, Spica Prunellae Vulgaris is commonly combined with Bulbus Fritillariae Thunbergii (*Zhe Bei Mu*) and Concha Ostreae (*Mu Li*).

Dosage: 10-15g

---

[4] Chinese texts often simply use the term *Zhu Ye*, Folium Bambusae, when identifying this medicinal.

Method of use: Decoct in water and administer internally.

Contraindications: Use cautiously in those with spleen-stomach vacuity weakness conditions.

Rhizoma Phragmitis Communis (*Lu Gen*)

Nature & flavor: Sweet and cold

Channel entry: Lungs and stomach

Functions: Clears heat and engenders fluids, eliminates vexation, stops vomiting, disinhibits urination

Indications:

1. Used for heat damaging fluids with high fever and thirst, Rhizoma Phragmitis Communis is commonly combined with Gypsum Fibrosum (*Shi Gao*) and Rhizoma Anemarrhenae Aspheloidis (*Zhi Mu*). For the treatment of vexation, thirst, and vomiting due to stomach heat, Rhizoma Phragmitis Communis can be combined with Caulis Bambusae In Taeniis (*Zhu Ru*) and uncooked Rhizoma Zingiberis (*Sheng Jiang*).

2. Used for lung abscess with coughing of phlegm with bloody threads, Rhizoma Phragmitis Communis can be combined with Semen Coicis Lachryma-jobi (*Yi Yi Ren*) and Semen Benincasae Hispidae (*Dong Gua Zi*).

Semen Cassiae Torae (*Jue Ming Zi*)

Nature & flavor: Sweet, bitter, and slightly cold

Channel entry: Liver and kidneys

Functions: Clears heat and brightens the eyes, moistens the intestines and frees the flow of the stool

Indications:

1. Used for redness and pain of the eyes due to either liver fire or wind heat, Semen Cassiae Torae is commonly combined with Flos Chrysanthemi Morifolii (*Ju Hua*). For the treatment of dizziness, photophobia, and blurred vision due to liver-kidney dual vacuity, Semen Cassiae Torae can be combined with Spica Prunellae Vulgaris (*Xia Ku Cao*).

2. Used for blood vacuity fluid dryness constipation, Semen Cassiae Torae is commonly combined with Radix Angelicae Sinensis (*Dang Gui*). If stomach heat has damaged fluids resulting in constipation with bad breath, red eyes, and reddish, scanty urination, Semen Cassiae Torae can be combined with Herba Lophatheri Gracilis (*Dan Zhu Ye*) and Semen Trichosanthis Kirlowii (*Gua Lou Ren*).

Dosage: 10-15g

Method of use: Decoct in water and administer internally.

B. Heat-clearing, dampness-drying medicinals

The natures and flavors of medicinals in this category are mostly bitter and cold and their action is to clear heat and dry dampness. They are mainly used for vexatious heat, a bitter taste in the mouth, slimy tongue fur, chest glomus, jaundice, diarrhea and dysentery, yellowish red urination, welling abscess swelling, sores, and toxins, joint swelling and pain, eczema, and other such damp heat conditions.

Radix Scutellariae Baicalensis (*Huang Qin*)

Nature & flavor: Bitter and cold

Channel entry: Lungs, gallbladder, stomach, and large intestine

Functions: Clears heat and dries dampness, drains fire and resolves toxins, stops bleeding, quiets the fetus

Indications:

1. Used for many types of damp heat patterns. In the treatment of damp warm fever, chest oppression, and slimy tongue fur, Radix Scutellariae Baicalensis is commonly combined with Talcum (*Hua Shi*) and Medulla Tetrapancis Papyriferi (*Tong Cao*) as in *Huang Qin Hua Shi Tang* (Scutellaria & Talcum Decoction). For damp heat jaundice, it is commonly combined with Fructus Gardeniae Jasminoidis (*Zhi Zi*) and Herba Artemisiae Capillaris (*Yin Chen Hao*). For the treatment of lower burner damp heat with astringent, painful urination, Radix Scutellariae Baicalensis is commonly combined with uncooked Radix Rehmanniae (*Sheng Di*) and Medulla Tetrapanacis Papyriferi (*Tong Cao*) as in *Huo Fu Dan* (Fire Mansion Elixir). For the treatment of welling abscesses, swelling, sores, and toxins, it is commonly combined with Radix Trichosanthis Kirlowii (*Tian Hua Fen*) and Radix Angelicae Dahuricae (*Bai Zhi*).

2. Used for acute heat diseases with symptoms of high fever, vexation and agitation, yellow tongue fur, and a rapid pulse, Radix Scutellariae Baicalensis is commonly combined with Rhizoma Coptidis Chinensis (*Huang Lian*) and Fructus Gardeniae Jasminoidis (*Zhi Zi*) as in *Huang Lian Jie Du Tang* (Coptis Resolve Toxins Decoction). If there is alternating hot and cold, Radix Scutellariae Baicalensis is commonly combined with Radix Bupleuri (*Chai Hu*) as in *Xiao Chai Hu Tang* (Minor Bupleurum Decoction).

3. Used for lung heat cough with coughing and spitting of yellow phlegm, this medicinal is commonly combined with Cortex Radicis Mori Albi (*Sang Bai Pi*) and Tuber Ophiopogonis Japonici (*Mai Men Dong*) as in *Qing Fei Tang* (Clear the Lungs Decoction).

4. Used for heat exuberance forcing the blood to move frenetically spitting of blood, spontaneous ejection of blood, hemafecia, and flooding and leaking precipitation of blood, carbonized Radix Scutellariae Baicalensis may be used alone or may be combined with uncooked Radix Rehmanniae (*Sheng Di*) and Rhizoma Imperatae Cylindricae (*Bai Mao Gen*).

5. Used for fetal heat and fetal stirring restlessness, this medicinal is commonly combined with Radix Angelicae Sinensis (*Dang Gui*) and Rhizoma Atractylodis Macrocephalae (*Bai Zhu*) as in *Dang Gui San* (Dang Gui Powder).

Dosage: 3-12g

Method of use: Decoct in water and administer internally or take as powder or pills. To clear heat, one should use uncooked. To quiet the fetus, mostly use stir-fried. To stop bleeding, one should use stir-fried till carbonized.

Cautions & contraindications: This medicinal is contraindicated in spleen-stomach vacuity cold with scanty eating and loose stools.

Rhizoma Coptidis Chinensis (*Huang Lian*)

Nature & flavor: Bitter and cold

Channel entry: Heart, stomach, liver, gallbladder, and large intestine

Functions: Clears heat and dries dampness, drains fire and resolves toxins

Indications:

1. Used for large intestine damp heat with the symptoms of diarrhea, downward dysentery, and tenesmus, Rhizoma Coptidis Chinensis is commonly combined with Radix Auklandiae Lappae (*Mu Xiang*) as in *Xiang Lian Wan* (Auklandia & Coptis Pills). If there is diarrhea and dysentry with simultaneous bodily heat exterior pattern, one can combine Rhizoma Coptidis Chinensis with Radix Puerariae (*Ge Gen*), Radix Scutellariae Baicalensis (*Huang Qin*), and mix-fried Radix Glycyrrhizae (*Gan Cao*). This is then called *Ge Gen Qin Lian Tang* (Pueraria, Scutellaria & Coptis Decoction). For cold and heat bound together in the middle burner with symptoms of stomach duct and abdominal glomus and fullness, vomiting, and nausea, Rhizoma Coptidis Chinensis is commonly combined with Radix Scutellariae Baicalensis (*Huang Qin*) and Rhizoma Pinelliae Ternatae (*Ban Xia*) as in *Ban Xia Xie Xin Tang* (Pinellia Drain the Heart Decoction).

2. Used for acute heat disease, fire and heat accumulation and exuberance with symptoms of high fever, vexation and agitation, spirit clouding, and delirious speech, Rhizoma Coptidis Chinensis is commonly combined with Radix Scutellariae Baicalensis (*Huang Qin*) and Fructus Gardeniae Jasminoidis (*Zhi Zi*) as in *Huang Lian Jie Du Tang* (Coptis Resolve Toxins Decoction). In terms of heart fire hyperactivity and exuberance with vexation and agitation and insomnia or heat forcing the blood to move frenetically thus resulting in spitting of blood or spontaneous ejection of blood, Rhizoma Coptidis Chinensis is commonly combined with Radix Scutellariae Baicalensis (*Huang Qin*) and Gelatinum Corii Asini (*E Jiao*) as in *Huang Lian E Jiao Tang* (Coptis & Donkey Skin Glue Decoction).

3. Used for welling abscess, swelling, sores, and toxins, *ding* toxins internally vanquishing, ear and eye swelling and pain, sores engendered the mouth and on the tongue, damp sores and itching, one can both administer Rhizoma Coptidis Chinensis internally and use it externally.

Dosage: 2-10g. Externally, use a suitable amount.

Method of use: Decoct in water and administer internally or take as powder or pills. Add to the decoction later.

Cautions & contraindications: This ingredient is greatly bitter and greatly cold. It is, therefore, not appropriate to use excessively large doses or to administer it for enduring periods of time so as not to damage the spleen. Its use is contraindicated if there is no damp heat or replete fire.

Cortex Phellodendri (*Huang Bai*)

Nature & flavor: Bitter and cold

Channel entry: Kidneys, urinary bladder, and large intestine

Functions: Clears heat and dries dampness, drains fire and resolves toxins, clears and recedes or abates vacuity heat

Indications:

1. Used for many types of damp heat conditions. In the treatment of damp heat downward dysentry with symptoms of body heat, abdominal pain, diarrhea, pus and blood in the stools, and tenesmus, Cortex Phellodendri is commonly combined with Radix Pulsatillae Chinensis (*Bai Tou Weng*) Cortex Fraxini (*Qin Pi*) and Rhizoma Coptidis Chinensis (*Huang Lian*). This is then called *Bai Tou Weng Tang* (Pulsatilla Decoction). In the treatment of damp heat jaundice, Cortex Phellodendri is commonly combined with Fructus Gardeniae Jasminoidis (*Zhi Zi*). This is then called *Zhi Zi Huang Pi Tang* (Gardenia & Phellodendron Decoction). In the treatment of damp heat abnormal vaginal discharge which is yellow, thick, foul-smelling, and turbid, Cortex Phellodendri is commonly combined with Semen Euryalis Ferocis (*Qian Shi*), Semen Gingkonis Bilobae (*Bai Guo*), and Semen Plantaginis (*Che Qian Zi*) as in *Yi Huang Tang* (Change Yellow Decoction). For the treatment of damp heat pouring downward with swelling and pain of the foot and lower leg, Cortex Phellodendri is commonly combined with Rhizoma Atractylodis (*Cang Zhu*) and Radix Achyranthis Bidentatae (*Niu Xi*) as in *San Miao San* (Three Wonders Powder). For urinary tract infections with astringent, painful urination, it can be combined with Caulis Akebiae (*Mu Tong*) and Semen Plantaginis (*Che Qian Zi*) or other such urination-disinhibiting, freeing the flow of strangury medicinals.

2. Used for the swelling and toxins of sores, eczema, oral sores, hemorrhoidal swelling, and injury due to scalding water and burns, Cortex Phellodendri can be administered internally and applied externally depending on the signs and symptoms.

3. Used for yin vacuity fire effulgence with symptoms of tidal heat, bone-steaming, night sweats, and seminal emission, Cortex Phellodendri is combined with Rhizoma Anemarrhenae Aspheloidis (*Zhi Mu*) as in *Zhi Bai Di Huang Wan* (Anemarrhena & Phellodendron Rehmannia Pills).

Dosage: 2-10g. Externally, use a suitable amount.

Method of use: Decoct in water and administer internally or take as powder or pills. Internally, it is mostly used stir-fried in salt-water. Externally, the uncooked is mostly used.

Cautions & contraindications: Due to its being bitter and cold, this ingredient easily damages the stomach qi and is, therefore, contraindicated in spleen-stomach vacuity cold.

Radix Gentianae Scabrae (*Long Dan Cao*)

Nature & flavor: Bitter and cold

Channel entry: Liver and gallbladder

Functions: Clears heat and dries dampness, drains liver-gallbladder fire

Indications:

1. Used for damp heat jaundice, Radix Gentianae Scabrae is commonly combined with Herba Artemisiae Capillaris (*Yin Chen Hao*) and Fructus Gardeniae Jasminoidis (*Zhi Zi*). In terms of damp heat pouring downward with scrotal swelling, genital itching, and a thick, yellow vaginal discharge, Radix Gentianae Scabrae is commonly combined with Semen Plantaginis (*Che Qian Zi*) and Radix Sophorae Flavescentis (*Ku Shen*).

2. Used for liver-gallbladder replete fire with headache, head distention, red, swollen, painful eyes, rib-side pain, a bitter taste in the mouth, and deafness, Radix Gentianae Scabrae is commonly combined with Radix Scutellariae Baicalensis (*Huang Qin*), Fructus Gardeniae Jasminoidis (*Zhi Zi*), and Radix Bupleuri (*Chai Hu*) as in *Long Dan Xie Gan Tang* (Gentiana Drain the Liver Decoction).

3. Used for liver heat engendering wind with high fever which does not recede and fright inversion convulsions, Radix Gentianae Scabrae is commonly combined with Rhizoma Coptidis Chinensis (*Huang Lian*) and Ramulus Uncariae Cum Uncis (*Gou Teng*) as in *Ling Jing Wan* (Cool Fright Pills).

Dosage: 3-10g

Method of use: Decoct in water and administer internally or take as powder or pills.

Cautions & contraindications: It is not appropriate to use an excessively large amount of this medicinal and it is contraindicated in spleen-stomach vacuity cold.

Radix Sophorae Flavescentis (*Ku Shen*)

Nature & flavor: Bitter and cold

Channel entry: Liver, kidneys, large intestine, and small intestine

Functions: Clears heat and dries dampness, kills worms, disinhibits urination

Indications:

1. Used for damp sores and eczema or abnormal vaginal discharge, Radix Sophorae Flavescentis is commonly combined with Semen Cnidii Monnieri (*She Chuang Zi*) and Cortex Phellodendri (*Huang Bai*).

2. Used for damp heat diarrhea and dysentery, Radix Sophorae Flavescentis can be combined with Radix Auklandiae Lappae (*Mu Xiang*).

3. Used for water swelling due to damp heat in the lower burner accompanied by astringent, painful urination with scanty, reddish urine, Radix Sophorae Flavescentis can be combined with Sclerotium Poriae Cocos (*Fu Ling*).

Dosage: 3-10g

Method of use: Decoct in water and administer internally or use as a fumigation and wash externally.

Cortex Fraxini (*Qin Pi*)

Nature & flavor: Bitter, astringent, and cold

Channel entry: Large intestine, stomach, and liver

Functions: Clears heat, dries dampness, restrains and astringes, and brightens the eyes

Indications:

1. Used for damp heat diarrhea and dysentery, Cortex Fraxini is commonly combined with Radix Pulsatillae Chinensis (*Bai Tou Weng*) and Rhizoma Coptidis Chinensis (*Huang Lian*) as in *Bai Tou Weng Tang* (Pulsatilla Decoction).

2. Used for redness and swelling of the eyes, external visual obstruction and styes, Cortex Fraxini is commonly combined with Rhizoma Coptidis Chinensis (*Huang Lian*) and Herba Lophatheri Gracilis (*Dan Zhu Ye*).

Dosage: 6-12g

Method of use: Decoct in water and administer internally.

Cautions & contraindications: This medicinal is contraindicated in case of spleen-stomach vacuity cold conditions.

C. Heat-clearing, blood-cooling medicinals

The medicinals in this category are mostly bitter, sweet, salty, and cold ingredients which have the action of clearing and resolving heat evils in the constructive and blood divisions. They are mainly used for warm heat disease heat entering the constructive and blood with symptoms of a crimson tongue, vexation and agitation, spirit clouding, and delirious speech, blood heat frenetic movement resulting in spitting of blood, spontaneous ejection of blood, or blood heat emission of macules and emission of rashes.

If heat enters the constructive and blood, it easily damages yin and consumes fluids. Therefore, when heat disease has damaged yin, these medicinals can be combined with yin-enriching medicinals.

Cornu Rhinocerotis (*Xi Jiao*)[5]

Nature & flavor: Bitter, salty, and cold

Channel entry: Heart, liver, and kidneys

Functions: Cools the blood and stops bleeding, clears the heart and quiets the spirit, resolves toxins and transforms macules

Indications:

1. Used for blood heat frenetic movement spitting of blood and spontaneous ejection of blood, Cornu Rhinocerotis is commonly combined with uncooked Radix Rehmanniae

---

[5] This medicinal is from a severely endangered species and should never be used as medicine. It can be replaced by Cornu Bubali (*Shui Niu Jiao*), water buffalo horn, of which there is no lack.

(*Sheng Di*), Radix Rubrus Paeoniae Lactiflorae (*Chi Shao*), and Cortex Radicis Moutan (*Dan Pi*) as in *Xi Jiao Di Huang Tang* (Rhinoceros Horn & Rehmannia Decoction).

2. Used for acute heat diseases with heat entering the heart constructive, strong fever which does not recede, clouding of the spirit, and delirious speech, Cornu Rhinocerotis is commonly combined with uncooked Radix Rehmanniae (*Sheng Di*), Radix Scrophulariae Ningpoensis (*Xuan Shen*), and Fructus Forsythiae Suspensae (*Lian Qiao*) as in *Qing Ying Tang* (Clear the Constructive Decoction). When used to treat heat falling into the heart and liver with high fever, vexation and agitation, and fright inversion convulsions, Cornu Rhinocerotis is commonly combined with Cornu Antelopis Saiga-tatarici (*Ling Yang Jiao*) as in *Zi Xue Dan* (Purple Snow Elixir).

3. Used for warm heat disease with heat toxins blazing and exuberant, body heat, and emission of macules, or emission of rash which is purple and dark in color, Cornu Rhinocerotis is commonly combined with Gypsum Fibrosum (*Shi Gao*) and Radix Scrophulariae Ningpoensis (*Xuan Shen*), as in *Hua Ban Tang* (Transform Macules Decoction).

Dosage: 1.5-6g

Method of use: File into fine powder and wash down with the decoction. It is also possible to decoct in water first and then add this decoction to the other medicinals as they decoct. Cornu Rhinocerotis may also be taken as powder or pills.

Cautions & contraindications: Cornu Rhinocerotis fears Radix Ligustici Wallichii (*Chuan Xiong*) and Radix Aconiti (*Cao Wu*). It should be used with care in pregnant women.

Uncooked Radix Rehmanniae (*Sheng Di*)

Nature & flavor: Sweet, bitter, and cold

Channel entry: Heart, liver, and kidneys

Functions: Clears heat and cools the blood, nourishes yin and engenders fluids

Indications:

1. Used for warm heat disease with heat entering the constructive and blood with symptoms of body heat, dry mouth, and a red or crimson tongue, uncooked Radix Rehmanniae is commonly combined with Cornu Rhinocerotis (*Xi Jiao*) and Radix

Scrophulariae Ningpoensis (*Xuan Shen*) as in *Qing Ying Tang* (Clear the Constructive Decoction).

2. Used for blood heat frenetically moving spitting of blood, spontaneous ejection of blood, hematuria, and flooding and leaking precipitation of blood, uncooked Radix Rehmanniae is commonly combined with Cacumen Biotae Orientalis (*Ce Bai Ye*), Folium Nelumbinis Nuciferae (*Ou Ye*), and Folium Artemisiae Argyii (*Ai Ye*) as in *Si Sheng Wan* (Four Uncooked [Ingredients] Pills). For the treatment of heat toxins blazing and exuberant with purplish black macules and rashes, it can be combined with Cornu Rhinocerotis (*Xi Jiao*) and Cortex Radicis Moutan (*Dan Pi*) as in *Xi Jiao Di Huang Tang* (Rhinoceros Horn & Rehmannia Decoction).

3. Used for the latter stage of heat disease with low-grade fever which does not abate or chronic disease with yin vacuity fever, uncooked Radix Rehmanniae is commonly combined with Radix Artemisiae Apiaceae (*Qing Hao*), Carapax Amydae Sinensis (*Bie Jia*) and Rhizoma Anemarrhenae Aspheloidis (*Zhi Mu*) as in *Qing Hao Bie Jia Tang* (Artemisia Apiacea & Carapax Amydae Decoction).

4. Used for heat disease which has damaged yin or yin vacuity wasting and thirsting. If heat disease has damaged yin with symptoms of oral thirst, a dry mouth, a red tongue, and dry lips, uncooked Radix Rehmanniae is commonly combined with Tuber Ophiopogonis Japonici (*Mai Men Dong*) and Radix Glehniae Littoralis (*Sha Shen*) as in *Yi Wei Tang* (Boost the Stomach Decoction). If exuberant heat has damaged yin with fluid depletion constipation, one can combine uncooked Radix Rehmanniae with Radix Scrophulariae Ningpoensis (*Xuan Shen*) and Tuber Ophiopogonis Japonici (*Mai Men Dong*) as in *Zeng Ye Tang* (Increase Humors Decoction). For wasting and thirsting with oral thirst and polydipsia, uncooked Radix Rehmanniae is commonly combined with Radix Puerariae (*Ge Gen*) and Radix Trichosanthis Kirlowii (*Tian Hua Fen*) as in *Yu Quan San* (Jade Spring Powder).

Dosage: 10-30g

Method of use: Decoct in water and administer internally. For clearing heat and engendering fluids, use uncooked. For stopping bleeding, use stir-fried till carbonized.

Cautions & contraindications: This ingredient is sweet, cold, and stagnating. Therefore, if the spleen has dampness with abdominal fullness and loose stools, this medicinal is contraindicated.

Radix Scrophulariae Ningpoensis (*Xuan Shen*)

Nature & flavor: Bitter, sweet, salty, and cold

Channel entry: Lungs, stomach, and kidneys

Functions: Clears heat and nourishes yin, drains fire and resolves toxins

Indications:

1. Used for warm heat disease with heat entering the constructive division with symptoms of body heat, oral thirst, vexation and agitation, restlessness, spirit clouding, and delirious speech, Radix Scrophulariae Ningpoensis is commonly combined with uncooked Radix Rehmanniae (*Sheng Di*), Cornu Rhinocerotis (*Xi Jiao*), and Fructus Forsythiae Suspensae (*Lian Qiao*) as in *Qing Ying Tang* (Clear the Constructive Decoction) and *Qing Gong Tang* (Clear the Palace Decoction). When used to treat heat toxins blazing and exuberant with emission of macules and rashes, it can be combined with Gypsum Fibrosum (*Shi Gao*), Cornu Rhinocerotis (*Xi Jiao*), and Rhizoma Anemarrhenae Aspheloidis (*Zhi Mu*) as in *Hua Ban Tang* (Transform Macules Decoction).

2. Used for throat swelling and pain, scrofulous phlegm kernels, or sloughing flat abscesses. For throat swelling and pain categorized as external contraction wind heat, Radix Scrophulariae Ningpoensis is commonly combined with Fructus Arctii Lappae (*Niu Bang Zi*) and Herba Menthae Haplocalycis (*Bo He*). When categorized as internal heat attacking upward, Radix Scrophulariae Ningpoensis is commonly combined with Tuber Ophiopogonis Japonici (*Mai Dong*), Radix Platycodi Grandiflori (*Jie Geng*), and Radix Glycyrrhizae (*Gan Cao*). This is then called *Xuan Mai Gan Jie Tang* (Scrophularia, Ophiopogon, Licorice & Platycodon Decoction). For scrofulous phlegm kernels, it is commonly combined with Bulbus Fritillariae (*Bei Mu*) and Concha Ostreae (*Mu Li*) as in *Xiao Luo Wan* (Disperse Scrofula Pills).

For sloughing flat abscesses, Radix Scrophulariae Ningpoensis is commonly combined with Flos Lonicerae Japonicae (*Jin Yin Hua*) and Radix Angelicae Sinensis (*Dang Gui*) as in *Si Miao Yong An Tang* (Fours Wonders Resting Hero Decoction).

Dosage: 10-15g

Method of use: Decoct in water and administer internally or take in powders or pills.

Cautions & contraindications: This medicinal is contraindicated in cases of spleen-stomach vacuity cold with scanty eating and loose stools. It reverses or opposes Radix Et Rhizoma Veratri (*Li Lu*).

Cortex Radicis Moutan (*Dan Pi*)

Nature & flavor: Bitter, acrid, and slightly cold

Channel entry: Heart, liver, and kidneys

Functions: Clears heat and cools the blood, quickens the blood and scatters stasis

Indications:

1. Used for warm heat disease heat entering the blood division with emission of macules and rashes and blood heat frenetically moving resulting in spitting of blood and spontaneous ejection of blood, Cortex Radicis Moutan is commonly combined with uncooked Radix Rehmanniae (*Sheng Di*) and Cornu Rhinocerotis (*Xi Jiao*) as in *Xi Jiao Di Huang Tang* (Rhinoceros Horn & Rehmannia Decoction).

2. Used for the latter stage of heat disease with heat deep-lying in the yin division, heat at night and coolness in the morning, and yin vacuity internal heat conditions, Cortex Radicis Moutan is commonly combined with Radix Artemisiae Apiaceae (*Qing Hao*) and Carapax Amydae Sinensis (*Bie Jia*) as in *Qing Hao Bie Jia Tang* (Artemisia Apiacea & Carapax Amydae Decoction). It can also be used for women's early menstruation and premenstrual fever. In that case, it is commonly combined with Radix Albus Paeoniae Lactiflorae (*Bai Shao*) and Radix Scutellariae Baicalensis (*Huang Qin*) as in *Xuan Yu Tong Jing Tang* (Diffuse Depression & Free the Flow of the Channels Decoction).

3. Used for blood stasis blocked menstruation, painful menstruation, or lumps within the abdomen, Cortex Radicis Moutan is commonly combined with Ramulus Cinnamomi Cassiae (*Gui Zhi*) and Semen Pruni Persicae (*Tao Ren*) as in *Gui Zhi Fu Ling Wan* (Cinnamon Twig & Poria Pills).

4. Used for intestinal abscess or abscesses, swellings, sores, and toxins. For intestinal abscesses with abdominal pain and constipation, Cortex Radicis Moutan is commonly combined with Radix Et Rhizoma Rhei (*Da Huang*) and Semen Pruni Persicae (*Tao Ren*) as in *Da Huang Mu Dan Pi Tang* (Rhubarb & Moutan Decoction). In terms of abscesses, swellings, sores, and toxins, it is commonly combined with Flos Lonicerae Japonicae (*Jin Yin Hua*), Fructus Forsythiae Suspensae (*Lian Qiao*), and Radix Angelicae Dahuricae (*Bai Zhi*).

Dosage: 6-12g

Method of use: Decoct in water and administer internally or take in powders or pills. To clear heat and cool the blood, use uncooked. To quicken the blood and scatter stasis, use stir-fried in alcohol. To stop bleeding, use stir-fried till carbonized.

Radix Rubrus Paeoniae Lactiflorae (*Chi Shao*)

Nature & flavor: Bitter and slightly cold

Channel entry: Liver

Functions: Clears heat and cools the blood, scatters stasis and stops pain

Indications:

1. Used for warm heat disease heat entering the blood division with body heat, emission of macules, and emission of rashes or blood heat frenetically moving spitting of blood and spontaneous ejection of blood, Radix Rubrus Paeoniae Lactiflorae is commonly combined with Cornu Rhinocerotis (*Xi Jiao*), uncooked Radix Rehmanniae (*Sheng Di*), and Cortex Radicis Moutan (*Dan Pi*) as in *Xi Jiao Di Huang Tang* (Rhinoceros Horn & Rehmannia Decoction).

2. Used for blood stasis blocked menstruation and painful menstruation, Radix Rubrus Paeoniae Lactiflorae is commonly combined with Radix Angelicae Sinensis (*Dang Gui*) and Cortex Radicis Moutan (*Dan Pi*) as in *Zi Xue Tang* (Enrich the Blood Decoction).

3. Used for liver heat red, swollen, painful eyes, welling abcess swelling, and clove sore toxins. For the former, Radix Rubrus Paeoniae Lactiflorae is commonly combined with Flos Chrysanthemi Morifolii (*Ju Hua*) and Herba Equiseti Hiemalis (*Mu Zei Cao*). For the latter, it is commonly combined with Flos Lonicerae Japonicae (*Jin Yin Hua*) and Rhizoma Coptidis Chinensis (*Huang Lian*) as in *Duo Ming Dan* (Destiny-clutching Elixir).

In addition, when this medicinal is combined with Semen Pruni Persicae (*Tao Ren*) and Flos Carthami Tinctorii (*Hong Hua*), it can treat swelling and pain due to external injury.

Dosage: 6-12g

Method of use: Decoct in water and administer internally.

Radix Lithospermi Seu Arnebiae (*Zi Cao*)

Nature & flavor: Sweet, salty, and cold

Channel entry: Pericardium, heart, and liver

Functions: Clears heat and cools the blood, quickens the blood, resolves toxins and out-thrusts rashes, moistens the intestines and frees the flow of the stool

Indications:

1. Used for dark purplish rashes from severe fire toxins, Radix Lithospermi Seu Arnebiae can be combined with Folium Daqingye (*Da Qing Ye*).

2. For welling abscesses due to severe internal fire toxins accompanied by constipation, Radix Lithospermi Seu Arnebiae can be combined with Semen Trichosanthis Kirlowii (*Gua Lou Ren*).

3. Used for warm heat disease non-smooth or uneasy emission of rash, Radix Lithospermi Seu Arnebiae can be combined with Fructus Forsythiae Suspensae (*Lian Qiao*).

4. Used for injury to the muscles and skin due to burns and scalds, Radix Lithospermi Seu Arnebiae may be combined with Radix Angelicae Sinensis (*Dang Gui*), sesame oil, and lard to make a paste for external application as in *Zi Cao Gao* (Lithospermum Paste).

Dosage: 4.5-10g. Externally, use a suitable amount.

Method of use: Decoct in water and administer internally, or boil in oil until the medicinals turn black, remove the dregs, add lard to stiffen, and apply externally.

Cortex Radicis Lycii Chinensis (*Di Gu Pi*)

Nature & flavor: Sweet and cold

Channel entry: Lungs, liver, and kidneys

Functions: Cools the blood and eliminates steaming, clears the lungs and downbears fire

Indications:

1. Used for steaming bones and tidal heat, Cortex Radicis Lycii Chinensis is commonly combined with Radix Stellariae Dichotomae (*Yin Chai Hu*).

2. Used for blood heat frenetic movement resulting in spitting of blood, spontaneous ejection of blood, static macules, and excessively profuse menstruation, Cortex Radicis Lycii Chinensis is commonly combined with Cortex Radicis Moutan (*Dan Pi*).

3. Used for genital itching when decocted and made into a wash with Semen Cnidii Monnieri (*She Chuang Zi*), Fructus Schisandrae Chinensis (*Wu Wei Zi*), and Herba Menthae Haplocalycis (*Bo He*).

Dosage: 10-15g

Method of administration: Decoct in water and administer internally or use externally as a wash.

Cautions & contraindications: This medicinal is contraindicated for use in spleen-stomach vacuity cold and exterior pattern conditions.

Radix Cynanchi Atrati (*Bai Wei*)

Nature & flavor: Bitter, salty, and cold

Channel entry: Lungs, stomach, and kidneys

Functions: Clears heat and cools the blood, disinhibits urination and frees the flow of strangury, resolves toxins and cures sores

Indications:

1. Used for warm evils damaging the constructive fever, yin vacuity fever, bone-steaming taxation heat, and postpartum blood vacuity fever, Radix Cynanchi Atrati is commonly combined with Cortex Radicis Lycii Chinensis (*Di Gu Pi*).

2. Used for vacuity heat resulting in blood heat frenetic movement hot strangury and bloody strangury, Radix Cynanchi Atrati can be combined with Herba Lophatheri Gracilis (*Dan Zhu Ye*) and/or Semen Plantaginis (*Che Qian Zi*).

3. Used for women's urinary incontinence with lack of knowledge at the time of exit, Radix Cynanchi Atrati can be combined with Radix Albus Paeonia Lactiflorae (*Bai Shao*).

4. Used for lung repletion nasal congestion, Radix Cynanchi Atrati can be combined with Radix Stemonae (*Bai Bu*), Flos Tussilaginis Farfarae (*Kuan Dong Hua*), and Bulbus Fritillariae (*Bei Mu*).

Dosage: 4.5-10g

Method of use: Decoct in water and administer internally.

Radix Stellariae Dichotomae (*Yin Chai Hu*)

Nature & flavor: Sweet and slightly cold

Channel entry: Liver and stomach

Functions: Clears vacuity heat, eliminates *gan* heat

Indications:

1. Used for blood vacuity steaming-bones with recurrent afternoon fever, spitting of blood, spontaneous ejection of blood, or flooding and leaking, Radix Stellariae Dichotomae can be combined with Rhizoma Picrorrhizae (*Hu Huang Lian*).

2. Used for chronic pediatric gan condition with fever, Radix Stellariae Dichotomae can be combined with Fructus Gardeniae Jasminoidis (*Zhi Zi*).

Dosage: 3-10g

Method of use: Decoct in water and administer internally.

Cautions & contraindications: This medicinal is contraindicated in case of external contraction of wind cold.

D. Heat-clearing, toxin-resolving medicinals

The medicinals in this category have the action of clearing fire heat and dispersing swellings and toxins. They are mainly used for warm heat diseases, sores and welling abscesses, cinnabar toxins, macules and rashes, throat swelling and pain, mumps, dysentery, and other such heat toxins disease conditions.

Flos Lonicerae Japonicae (*Jin Yin Hua*)

Nature & flavor: Sweet and cold

Channel entry: Lungs, stomach, and large intestine

Functions: Clears heat and resolves toxins, cools the blood and stops dysentery

Indications:

1. Used for external contraction wind heat or the initial stage of warm heat disease with symptoms of fever, slight aversion to wind and cold, etc., Flos Lonicerae Japonicae is commonly combined with Fructus Forsythiae Suspensae (*Lian Qiao*) and Herba Menthae Haplocalycis (*Bo He*) as in *Yin Qiao San* (Lonicera & Forsythia Powder).

2. Used for heat entering the qi division with symptoms of strong fever, vexatious thirst, and a surging, large pulse, Flos Lonicerae Japonicae is commonly combined with Gypsum Fibrosum (*Shi Gao*) and Rhizoma Anemarrhenae Aspheloidis (*Zhi Mu*).

3. Used for sores and welling abscesses. This ingredient is a commonly used, main medicinal in the external medicine department. It is commonly combined with Herba Taraxaci Mongolici Cum Radice (*Pu Gong Ying*) and Herba Violae Yedoensitis Cum Radice (*Zi Hua Di Ding*) as in *Wu Wei Xiao Du Yin* (Five Flavors Disperse Toxins Drink).

4. Used for heat toxins diarrhea and dysentery with downward precipitation of pus and blood, Flos Lonicerae Japonicae is commonly combined with Radix Scutellariae Baicalensis (*Huang Qin*), Rhizoma Coptidis Chinensis (*Huang Lian*), and Radix Pulsatillae Chinensis (*Bai Tou Weng*). It may also be used alone as a thick decoction which is then drunk frequently.

Dosage: 10-15g. For heat exuberance and heavy toxins, one can use up to 30-60g.

Method of use: Decoct in water and administer internally.

Note: Caulis Lonicerae Japonicae (*Ren Dong Teng*) has the same actions as Flos Lonicerae Japonicae and also clears wind heat from the channels and network vessels. It is commonly used for welling abscess swelling, sores, and toxins, swollen, painful throat, and red, swollen, hot, painful joints, *i.e.*, wind damp heat impediment pain. Its dosage is 15-30g.

Fructus Forsythiae Suspensae (*Lian Qiao*)

Nature & flavor: Bitter and slightly cold

Channel entry: Lungs, heart, and gallbladder

Functions: Clears heat and resolves toxins, disperses swelling and scatters nodulations

Indications:

1. Used for external contraction wind heat or the initial stage of a warm disease with symptoms of fever, headache, oral thirst, etc., Fructus Forsythiae Suspensae is commonly combined with Flos Lonicerae Japonicae (*Jin Yin Hua*) as in *Yin Qiao San* (Lonicera & Forsythia Powder). If there is heat entering the pericardium with high fever, vexation and agitation, and spirit clouding, Fructus Forsythiae Suspensae is commonly combined with Cornu Rhinocerotis (*Xi Jiao*) and Plumula Nelumbinis Nuciferae (*Lian Zi Xin*) as in *Qing Gong Tang* (Clear the Palace Decoction).

2. Used for heat toxins brewing and binding resulting in various types of abscesses, swellings, and sores or scrofulous bindings and kernels. This ingredient is a main medicinal for sores. In the treatment of abscesses, swellings, and sores, it is commonly combined with Flos Lonicerae Japonicae (*Jin Yin Hua*) and Herba Taraxaci Mongolici Cum Radice (*Pu Gong Ying*). In the treatment of scrofulous bindings and kernels, it is commonly combined with Spica Prunellae Vulgaris (*Xia Ku Cao*) and Bulbus Fritillariae (*Bei Mu*).

Dosage: 6-15g

Method of use: Decoct in water and administer internally.

Folium Daqingye (*Da Qing Ye*)

Nature & flavor: Bitter and greatly cold

Channel entry: Heart, lungs, and stomach

Functions: Clears heat and resolves toxins, cools the blood and disperses macules

Indications:

1. Used for warm heat disease heat entering the blood division with strong fever, vexation and agitation, emission of macules and rashes, spirit clouding, and delirium, Folium

Daqingye is commonly combined with Cornu Rhinocerotis (*Xi Jiao*) and Fructus Gardeniae Jasminoidis (*Zhi Zi*) as in *Xi Jiao Da Qing Tang* (Rhinoceros Horn & Isatis Decoction). When used to treat external contraction wind heat or the initial stage of a warm heat disease with fever, headache, and oral thirst, it can be combined with Flos Lonicerae Japonicae (*Jin Yin Hua*) and Fructus Arctii Lappae (*Niu Bang Zi*).

2. Used for blood heat toxin exuberance cinnabar toxins, oral sores, and throat swelling and pain, Folium Daqingye is commonly combined with Flos Lonicerae Japonicae (*Jin Yin Hua*) and Radix Scrophulariae Ningpoensis (*Xuan Shen*).

Dosage: 10-15g

Method of use: Decoct in water and administer internally.

Radix Isatidis Seu Baphicacanthi (*Ban Lan Gen*)

Nature & flavor: Bitter and cold

Channel entry: Heart and stomach

Functions: Clears heat and resolves toxins, cools the blood and disinhibits the throat

Indications:

1. Used for warm heat disease with fever and headache or big head epidemic toxins with red, swollen face and head, inhibited throat, ulcerated throat, or cinnabar sand, Radix Isatidis Seu Baphicacanthi is commonly combined with Fructus Forsythiae Suspensae (*Lian Qiao*) and Radix Scrophulariae Ningpoensis (*Xuan Shen*) as in *Pu Ji Xiao Du Yin* (*Universal Relief* Disperse Toxins Drink).

2. Used for the initial stage of a warm disease or external contraction wind heat with fever, headache, oral thirst, etc., it can be combined with Flos Lonicerae Japonicae (*Jin Yin Hua*) and Fructus Forsythiae Suspensae (*Lian Qiao*).

In addition, this medicinal is commonly used in clinic for the treatment of influenza.

Dosage: 10-15g

Method of use: Decoct in water and administer internally.

Radix Pulsatillae Chinensis (*Bai Tou Weng*)

Nature & flavor: Bitter and cold

Channel entry: Large intestine

Functions: Clears heat and resolves toxins, cools the blood and stops dysentery

Indications: Used for the treatment of heat toxins diarrhea and dysentery, red dysentery with abdominal pain, and tenesmus, this ingredient has very good treatment efficacy for both bacterial and amebic dysentery. It is commonly combined with Cortex Phellodendri (*Huang Bai*), Rhizoma Coptidis Chinensis (Huang *Lian*), and Cortex Fraxini (*Qin Pi*) as in *Bai Tou Weng Tang* (Pulsatilla Decoction).

In addition, when this ingredient is used together with Radix Sophorae Flavescentis (*Ku Shen*) as an external wash, it can treat vaginal tract trichomoniasis.

Dosage: 6-15g. Externally, use a suitable amount.

Method of use: Decoct in water and administer internally.

Herba Taraxaci Mongolici Cum Radice (*Pu Gong Ying*)

Nature & flavor: Bitter, sweet, and cold

Channel entry: Liver and stomach

Functions: Clears heat and resolves toxins, disperses swelling and scatters nodulations, disinhibits urination and frees the flow of strangury

Indications:

1. Used for breast abscesses, welling and flat abscesses, Herba Taraxaci Mongolici Cum Radice is commonly combined with Fructus Trichosanthis Kirlowii (*Gua Lou*), Bulbus Fritillariae Thunbergii (*Zhe Bei Mu*), and Resina Myrrhae (*Mo Yao*). Used for various types of hard, hot, painful welling abscesses and clove sores, Herba Taraxaci Mongolici Cum Radice can be combined with Flos Lonicerae Japonicae (*Jin Yin Hua*) and Fructus Forsythiae Suspensae (*Lian Qiao*).

2. Used for redness and swelling of the eyes due to depressive heat in the stomach and liver channels, Herba Taraxaci Mongolici can be combined with Flos Chrysanthemi Morifolii (*Ju Hua*) and Radix Scutellariae Baicalensis (*Huang Qin*).

3. Used for scrofulous phlegm kernels, Herba Taraxaci Mongolici Cum Radice can be combined with Spica Prunellae Vulgaris (*Xia Ku Cao*).

In addition, the fresh herb may be pounded and mashed and applied externally to red, hot, swollen sores, and a wash made from a decoction of this medicinal maybe used externally for various types of sores and damp hot skin lesions as well as for inflammation of the genitals.

Dosage: 9-15g. This medicinal may be used in large doses of up to 30-60g. Externally, use a suitable amount.

Method of use: Decoct in water and administer internally or as an external wash, or pound the fresh herb and apply externally to the affected area.

Herba Violae Yedoensitis Cum Radice (*Zi Hua Di Ding*)

Nature & flavor: Bitter, acrid, and cold

Channel entry: Heart and liver

Functions: Clears heat and resolves toxins, cools the blood and disperses swelling

Indications: Used for clove sores and welling abscess swelling and toxins, cinnabar toxins, welling and flat abscesses emitted on the upper back, Herba Violae Yedoensitis Cum Radice is commonly combined with Flos Lonicerae Japonicae (*Jin Yin Hua*), Fructus Forsythiae Suspensae (*Lian Qiao*), and Herba Taraxaci Mongolici Cum Radice (*Pu Gong Ying*).

Dosage: 15-30g. In larger doses, this medicinal can be used up to 30-60g. Externally, use a suitable amount.

Method of use: Decoct in water and administer internally or pound and mash the fresh herb and apply externally.

Herba Houttuyniae Cordatae Cum Radice (*Yu Xing Cao*)

Nature & flavor: Acrid and slightly cold

Channel entry: Lungs and liver

Functions: Clears heat and resolves toxins, disperses abscesses and expels pus, disinhibits urination and frees the flow of strangury

Indications:

1. Used for lung abscesses or lung heat cough with thick, yellow and green phlegm, Herba Houttuyniae Cordatae Cum Radice is commonly combined with Radix Platycodi Grandiflori (*Jie Geng*).

2. Used for welling abscess swelling and toxins due to replete heat, Herba Houttuyniae Cordatae Cum Radice is commonly combined with Flos Lonicerae Japonicae (*Jin Yin Hua*) and Herba Taraxaci Mongolici Cum Radice (*Pu Gong Ying*).

3. Used for damp heat astringent, painful urination and strangury, Herba Houttuyniae Cordatae Cum Radice can be combined with Semen Plantaginis (*Che Qian Zi*) and Rhizoma Imperatae Cylindricae (*Bai Mao Gen*).

4. Used for damp heat dysentery with pus and blood in the stools, Herba Houttuyniae Cordatae Cum Radice can be combined with Radix Pulsatillae Chinensis (*Bai Tou Weng*), Rhizoma Coptidis Chinensis (*Huang Lian*), and Herba Patriniae Heterophyllae Cum Radice (*Bai Jiang Cao*).

In addition, this medicinal when used fresh can be pounded and mashed and applied externally, the juice may be applied externally, or a decoction may be used to fumigate and wash the affected area.

Dosage: 15-30g. Externally, use a suitable amount.

Method of use: Decoct in water and administer or apply the macerated herb, its juice, or a decoction externally. It is not appropriate to decoct this medicinal for a long time and it is better to use the fresh herb.

Herba Patriniae Heterophyllae Cum Radice (*Bai Jiang Cao*)

Nature & flavor: Acrid, bitter, and slightly cold

Channel entry: Liver, stomach, and large intestine

Functions: Clears heat and resolves toxins, quickens the blood and dispels stasis

Indications:

1. Used for intestinal abscesses which have already transformed pus, Herba Patriniae Heterophyllae Cum Radice is commonly combined with Semen Coicis Lachryma-jobi (*Yi Yi Ren*) as in *Yi Yi Fu Zi Bai Jiang San* (Coix, Aconite & Patrinia Powder).

2. Used for damp heat stasis and stagnation lower abdominal pain and painful menstruation, especially on the right side, Herba Patriniae Hetrophyllae Cum Radice may be combined with Caulis Sargentodoxae (*Hong Teng*) and Radix Rubrus Paeoniae Lactiflorae (*Chi Shao*).

3. Used for damp heat dysentery and diarrhea with pus and blood in the stools, this medicinal may be combined with Herba Houttuyniae Cordatae Cum Radice (*Yu Xing Cao*), Radix Rubrus Paeoniae Lactiflorae (*Chi Shao*), and Rhizoma Coptidis Chinensis (*Huang Lian*).

Dosage: 10-30g

Method of use: Decoct in water and administer internally.

Cortex Radicis Dictamni Dasycarpi (*Bai Xian Pi*)

Nature & flavor: Bitter and cold

Channel entry: Spleen and stomach

Functions: Clears heat and dries dampness, dispels wind and resolves toxins

Indications:

1. Used for damp heat sores and toxins which drip yellow water, Cortex Radicis Dictamni Dasycarpi is commonly combined with Radix Sophorae Flavescentis (*Ku Shen*) and Semen Cnidii Monnieri (*She Chuang Zi*).

2. Used for wind rash, *i.e.*, hives, eczema, and itching, it is commonly combined with Radix Ledebouriellae Divaricatae (*Fang Feng*) and Fructus Tribuli Terrestris (*Bai Ji li*).

In addition, this ingredient can also be used to treat wind damp heat impediment and jaundice with reddish urine.

Dosage: 4.5-10g. Externally, use a suitable amount.

Method of use: Decoct in water and administer internally or apply to the affected area as a wash or powder.

Cautions & contraindications: This medicinal is not appropriate for use in vacuity cold conditions.

Rhizoma Smilacis Glabrae (*Tu Fu Ling*)

Nature & flavor: Sweet, bland, and level

Channel entry: Liver and stomach

Functions: Eliminates dampness, resolves toxins, frees the flow of and disinhibits the joints and sinews

Indications:

1. Used for damp heat impediment with aching and pain in the joints and sinews, Rhizoma Smilacis Glabrae can be combined with Semen Coicis Lachryma-jobi (*Yi Yi Ren*).

2. Used for turbid strangury due to damp heat toxins or vaginal discharge due to damp heat, Rhizoma Smilacis Glabrae can be combined with Rhizoma Dioscoreae Hypoglaucae (*Bei Xie*) and Rhizoma Acori Graminei (*Shi Chang Pu*).

3. Used for damp heat in the liver and gallbladder resulting in jaundice, Rhizoma Smilacis Glabrae can be combined with Herba Taraxaci Mongolici Cum Radice (*Pu Gong Ying*).

4. Used for damp heat sores and open sores, this medicinal can be combined with Cortex Radicis Dictamni Dasycarpi (*Bai Xian Pi*).

In addition, this medicinal can be used for plum toxins (*i.e.*, syphilis) or to treat mercury poisoning due to syphilis accompanied by spasms and contractures of the limbs and muscles.

Dosage: 15-60g. Externally, use a suitable amount.

Method of use: Decoct in water and administer internally or apply the decoction as a wash externally for genital inflammation and abnormal vaginal discharge.

Rhizoma Guanzhong (*Guan Zhong*)

Nature & flavor: Bitter and slightly cold. Has small toxins.

Channel entry: Liver and spleen

Functions: Clears heat and resolves toxins, expels worms, stops bleeding

Indications:

1. Used for intestinal parasites and abdominal pain, Rhizoma Guanzhong can be combined with Fructus Quisqualis Indicae (*Shi Jun Zi*), Fructificatio Polypori Mylittae (*Lei Wan*), and Semen Arecae Catechu (*Bing Lang*).

2. Used for epidemic big head wind, *i.e.*, mumps, and for sores and open sores due to heat toxins, Rhizoma Guanzhong is commonly combined with Flos Lonicerae Japonicae (*Jin Yin Hua*), Fructus Forsythiae Suspensae (*Lian Qiao*), and Herba Taraxaci Mongolici Cum Radice (*Pu Gong Ying*).

3. Used for blood heat women's flooding and leaking, Rhizoma Guanzhong can be combined with Cacumen Biotae Orientalis (*Ce Bai Ye*) and Radix Sanguisorbae (*Di Yu*).

Dosage: 3-10g

Method of use: Decoct in water and administer internally. For resolving toxins, use uncooked. For blood heat flooding and leaking, use stir-fried till carbonized.

E. Summerheat-resolving, heat-clearing medicinals

The medicinals in this category clear heat but are level or at most cool in nature rather than cold. They clear summerheat by upbearing the clear and downbearing the turbid, thus disinhibiting urination. At the same time, they engender fluids and stop thirst. They are mainly used for summerheat heat conditions with symptoms of fever, sweating, vexation, diarrhea, and thirst.

Folium Nelumbinis Nuciferae (*He Ye*)

Nature & flavor: Bitter and level

Channel entry: Heart, liver, and spleen

Functions: Clears heat and resolves summerheat, upbears and effuses clear yang, cools the blood and stops bleeding

Indications:

1. Used for summerheat heat vexatious thirst and summerheat dampness diarrhea especially when accompanied by spleen vacuity, Folium Nelumbinis Nuciferae is commonly combined with Semen Dolichoris Lablab (*Bai Bian Dou*).

2. Used for blood heat spitting of blood, spontaneous ejection of blood, hemafecia, and women's flooding and leaking, Folium Nelumbinis Nuciferae can be used alone, carbonized, powdered, and swallowed, or combined with Herba Cephalanoploris (*Xiao Ji*), Fructus Gardeniae Jasminoidis (*Zhi Zi*), Rhizoma Imperatae Cylindricae (*Bai Mao Gen*), and Cacumen Biotae Orientalis (*Ce Bai Ye*) as in *Shi Hui San* (Ten Ashed [Ingredients] Powder).

Semen Phaseoli Munginis (*Lu Dou*)

Nature & flavor: Sweet and cool

Channel entry: Heart and stomach

Functions: Clears summerheat and disinhibits urination

Indications: Used for summerheat vexatious thirst and fever, Semen Phaseoli Munginis can be used alone or may be combined with Rhizoma Coptidis Chinensis (*Huang Lian*) and Radix Glycyrrhizae (*Gan Cao*).

In addition, a thick decoction of large doses of this medicinal cooked with Radix Glycyrrhizae (*Gan Cao*) can be used to counteract the toxic side effects of Radix Lateralis Praeparatus Aconiti Carmichaeli (*Fu Zi*).

Dosage: 15-30g, and in large doses up to 120g.

Method of use: Decoct in water and administer internally or eat as soup.

Semen Dolichoris Lablab (*Bai Bian Dou*)

Nature & flavor: Sweet and level

Channel entry: Spleen and stomach

Functions: Harmonizes the stomach and disperses summerheat, fortifies the spleen and transforms dampness

Indications:

1. Used for brewing summerheat and dampness resulting in the arising of vomiting, diarrhea, chest oppression, abdominal distention, and devitalized eating and drinking, Semen Dolichoris Lablab is commonly combined with Herba Elsholtziae Splendentis (*Xiang Ru*) and Cortex Magnoliae Officinalis (*Hou Po*).

2. Used for spleen vacuity diarrhea and abnormal vaginal discharge, Semen Dolichoris Lablab is commonly combined with Radix Dioscoreae Oppositae (*Shan Yao*) and Rhizoma Atractylodis Macrocephalae (*Bai Zhu*).

Dosage: 10-15g

Method of use: Decoct in water and administer internally. For fortifying the spleen and transforming dampness, use stir-fried.

F. Vacuity heat clearing & receding medicinals

Medicinals in this category have the effect of cooling the blood and receding vacuity heat. They are mainly used for bone-steaming and tidal heat, heat in the hands, feet, and heart, night-time heat with morning coolness, or a low-grade fever which will not abate. They are commonly combined with yin-nourishing medicinals.

Herba Artemisiae Apiaceae (*Qing Hao*)

Nature & flavor: Bitter, slightly acrid, and cold

Channel entry: Liver, gallbladder, and kidneys

Functions: Cools the blood and recedes or abates steaming, clears the gallbladder and prevents the recurrence of malaria, clears heat and resolves summerheat

Indications:

1. Used for the latter stage of heat diseases with heat deep-lying in the yin division, night-time heat, morning coolness, or a low-grade fever which will not recede after a heat disease, Herba Artemisiae Apiaceae is commonly combined with Carapax Amydae Sinensis (*Bie Jia*) and uncooked Radix Rehmanniae (*Sheng Di*) as in *Qing Hao Bie Jia Tang* (Artemisia Apiacea & Carapax Amydae Decoction). In the treatment of yin vacuity bone-steaming and tidal heat, night sweats, and hand, foot, and heart heat, Herba Artemisiae Apiaceae can be combined with Radix Gentianae Macrophyllae (*Qin Jiao*) and Carapax Amydae Sinensis (*Bie Jia*) as in *Qin Jiao Bie Jia San* (Gentiana Macrophylla & Carapax Amydae Powder).

2. Used for the hot and cold of malaria-like disease, Herba Artemisiae Apiaceae is commonly combined with Radix Scutellariae Baicalensis (*Huang Qin*) and Rhizoma Pinelliae Ternatae (*Ban Xia*) as in *Hao Qin Qing Dan Tang* (Capillaris & Scutellaria Clear the Gallbladder Decoction).

3. Used for summerheat heat external contraction with fever, no sweating or possible sweating, dizziness, and headache, Herba Artemisiae Apiaceae is commonly combined with Talcum (*Hua Shi*) and Folium Nelumbinis Nuciferae (*Ou Ye*). It can also be used for pediatric summer-fall fever, in which case, it is commonly combined with Cortex Radicis Lycii Chinensis (*Di Gu Pi*) and Rhizoma Anemarrhenae Aspheloidis (*Zhi Mu*).

Dosage: 6-15g. In larger doses, this medicinal can be used in up to 18-30g.

Method of use: Decoct in water and administer internally. It is not appropriate to decoct this medicinal a long time.

Cortex Radicis Lycii Chinensis (*Di Gu Pi*)

Nature & flavor: Sweet and cold

Channel entry: Lungs and kidneys

Functions: Cools the blood and recedes steaming, clears and discharges lung heat

Indications:

1. Used for yin vacuity bone-steaming, tidal heat, night sweats, and pediatric gan fever, Cortex Radicis Lycii Chinensis is commonly combined with Rhizoma Anemarrhenae

Aspheloidis (*Zhi Mu*) and Carapax Amydae Sinensis (*Bie Jia*) as in *Di Gu Pi Tang* (Cortex Lycii Decoction).

2. Used for lung heat coughing and panting or coughing blood, Cortex Radicis Lycii Chinensis is commonly combined with Cortex Radicis Mori Albi (*Sang Bai Pi*) and Radix Glycyrrhizae (*Gan Cao*) as in *Xie Bai San* (Drain the White Powder).

In addition, when this medicinal is combined with Cacumen Biotae Orientalis (*Ce Bai Ye*) and Rhizoma Imperatae Cylindricae (*Bai Mao Gen*), it can be used for blood heat frenetic movement spitting of blood and spontaneous ejection of blood. When it is combined with Radix Trichosanthis Kirlowii (*Tian Hua Fen*) and uncooked Radix Rehmanniae (*Sheng Di*), it can treat the polyuria of wasting and thirsting.

Dosage: 6-15g

Method of use: Decoct in water and administer internally.

3

Phlegm-transforming, cough-stopping, panting-leveling medicinals

Medicinals whose action is to mainly dispel and eliminate phlegm turbidity are called phlegm-transforming medicinals. Those which are able to decrease or stop coughing and harmonize qi panting are called cough-stopping, panting-leveling medicinals. Since phlegm-transforming and cough-stopping, panting-leveling medicinals are mostly used together, therefore they are grouped together in this chapter. Phlegm-transforming medicinals are further divided into those which warm and transform cold phlegm and those which clear and transform hot phlegm. Phlegm-transforming medicinals are mainly used for profuse phlegm coughs, phlegm rheum qi panting, cough with phlegm which is difficult to expectorate, and other diseases due to phlegm, such as epilepsy, fright reversal, scrofula, and yin welling abscess flowing and pouring. Cough-stopping medicinals are mainly used for external contraction or internal damage resulting in coughing and panting respiration.

A. Cold phlegm warming & transforming medicinals

Rhizoma Pinelliae Ternatae (*Ban Xia*)

Nature & flavor: Acrid and warm. Has small toxins.

Channel entry: Spleen, stomach, and lungs

Functions: Dries dampness and transforms phlegm, downbears counterflow and stops vomiting, disperses glomus and scatters nodulations

Indications:

1. Used for spleen not transforming dampness and phlegm drool blockage and stagnation resulting in profuse phlegm, coughing, qi counterflow, and dizziness, Rhizoma Pinelliae Ternatae is commonly combined with Pericarpium Citri Reticulatae (*Chen Pi*) and Sclerotium Poriae Cocos (*Fu Ling*) as in *Er Chen Tang* (Two Aged [Ingredients] Decoction). If phlegm is profuse, clear, and watery tending to cold, Rhizoma Pinelliae Ternatae can be combined with Herba Asari Cum Radice (*Xi Xin*) and dry Rhizoma Zingiberis (*Gan Jiang*) or other lung-warming, rheum-transforming medicinals. If phlegm is thick in consistency and yellow in color tending to heat, Rhizoma Pinelliae Ternatae can

be combined with Radix Scutellariae Baicalensis (*Huang Qin*) and Fructus Trichosanthis Kirlowii (*Gua Lou*) or other heat-clearing, phlegm-transforming medicinals.

2. Used for stomach qi upward counterflow with nausea and vomiting. If there is cold rheum vomiting and spitting, Rhizoma Pinelliae Ternatae is commonly combined with uncooked Rhizoma Zingiberis (*Sheng Jiang*) as in *Xiao Ban Xia Tang* (Minor Pinellia Decoction). If there is stomach vacuity vomiting and spitting, it is mostly combined with Radix Panacis Ginseng (*Ren Shen*) and white honey as in *Da Ban Xia Tang* (Major Pinellia Decoction). If there is stomach heat vomiting and spitting, it can be combined with Rhizoma Coptidis Chinensis (*Huang Lian*) and Caulis Bambusae In Taeniis (*Zhu Ru*). For vomiting and spitting during pregnancy, it is commonly combined with Fructus Amomi (*Sha Ren*) and Caulis Perillae Frutescentis (*Su Gen*).

3. Used for chest and stomach duct glomus and oppression, plum pit qi, and scrofulous phlegm kernels, welling and flat abscesses, swellings and toxins. For the treatment of phlegm and heat mutually binding chest and venter glomus and oppression and vomiting, Rhizoma Pinelliae Ternatae is commonly combined with Rhizoma Coptidis Chinensis (*Huang Lian*) and Fructus Trichosanthis Kirlowii (*Gua Lou*) as in *Xiao Xian Xiong Tang* (Minor Fallen Chest Decoction). For the treatment of abnormal sensations in the region of the throat which cannot be discharged by spitting nor can be swallowed down, *i.e.*, plum pit qi, Rhizoma Pinelliae Ternatae is commonly combined with Cortex Magnoliae Offficinalis (*Hou Po*) and Folium Perillae Frutescentis (*Zi Su Ye*) as in *Ban Xia Hou Po Tang* (Pinellia & Magnolia Decoction). For the treatment of goiter and phlegm kernels, mostly Rhizoma Pinelliae Ternatae is combined with Thallus Algae (*Kun Bu*) and Herba Sargassii (*Hai Zao*). For the treatment of welling and flat abscesses on the upper back and breast sores, one can use powdered uncooked Rhizoma Pinelliae Ternatae mixed with egg whites and applied to the affected area.

Dosage: 3-10g

Method of use: Decoct in water and administer internally. Externally, use a suitable amount. Clear Rhizoma Pinelliae Ternatae is effective for transforming damp phlegm. Gingered Rhizoma Pinelliae Ternatae is good at stopping vomiting. Lime-processed is used to dry dampness and harmonize the stomach. Externally, it is the uncooked which is mostly used for welling and flat abscess swelling and toxins.

Cautions & contraindications: Reverses or opposes Radix Aconiti (*Wu Tou*).

Flos Inulae Racemosae (*Xuan Fu Hua*)

Nature & flavor: Bitter, acrid, salty, and slightly warm

Channel entry: Lungs, spleen, stomach, and large intestine

Functions: Disperses phlegm and moves water, downbears the qi and stops vomiting

Indications:

1. Used for phlegm rheum internally gathering resulting in chest and diaphragmatic glomus and oppression, Flos Inulae Racemosae is commonly combined with Radix Platycodi Grandiflori (*Jie Geng*) and Cortex Radicis Mori Albi (*Sang Bai Pi*) as in *Xuan Fu Hua Tang* (Inula Decoction). If there is external contraction cold evils with cough, phlegm, and panting, one can combine Flos Inulae Racemosae with Herba Asari Cum Radice (*Xi Xin*) and Rhizoma Pinelliae Ternatae (*Ban Xia*) as in *Jin Fei Cao San* (Inula Powder).

2. Used for spleen-stomach qi vacuity with phlegm dampness counterflowing upward glomus and fullness beneath the heart, vomiting and spitting, and burping, Flos Inulae Racemosae is commonly combined with Haemititum (*Dai Zhe Shi*) and Rhizoma Pinelliae Ternatae (*Ban Xia*) as in *Xuan Fu Dai Zhe Tang* (Inula & Hematite Decoction).

Dosage: 3-10g

Method of use: Decoct in water and administer internally. Wrap during decoction.

Semen Sinapis Albae (*Bai Jie Zi*)

Nature & flavor: Acrid and warm

Channel entry: Lungs and stomach

Functions: Sweeps phlegm and disinhibits the qi, scatters nodulations and disperses swelling

Indications:

1. Used for cold phlegm blocking the lungs with symptoms of cough, qi panting, and profuse, clear, watery phlegm, Semen Sinapis Albae is commonly combined with Fructus Perillae Frutescentis (*Zi Su Zi*) and Semen Raphani Sativi (*Lai Fu Zi*) as in *San Zi Yang Qin Tang* (Three Seeds Nourish the Aged Decoction). If there is phlegm rheum and qi counterflow with coughing and chest pain, and chest and rib-side accumulation of water,

one can combine Semen Sinapis Albae with Radix Euphorbiae Kansui (*Gan Sui*) and Radix Euphorbiae Seu Knoxiae (*Da Ji*) as in *Kong Xian Dan* (Controlling Drool Elixir).

2. Used for phlegm dampness flowing and pouring with yin flat abscess swelling and toxins, Semen Sinapis Albae is commonly combined with Gelatinum Cornu Cervi (*Lu Jiao Jiao*) and Cortex Cinnamomi Cassiae (*Rou Gui*) as in *Yang He Tang* (Yang-harmonizing Decoction).

In addition, this ingredient can be combined with Semen Momordicae Cochinensis (*Mu Bie Zi*) and Resina Myrrhae (*Mo Yao*) and prepared into powder for the treatment of phlegm stagnating in the channels and network vessels arm and shoulder aching, pain, and numbness.

Dosage: 3-10g. Externally, use a suitable amount.

Method of use: Decoct in water and administer internally.

Cautions & contraindications: Externally, this medicinal has a blistering action. Its use is contraindicated in those with skin allergies.

Rhizoma Arisaematis (*Tian Nan Xing*)

Nature & flavor: Bitter, acrid, and warm. Has toxins.

Channel entry: Lungs, liver, and spleen

Functions: Dries dampness and transforms phlegm, dispels wind and stops tetany, scatters nodulations and disperses swelling

Indications:

1. Used for damp phlegm chest and abdominal fullness and distention, cough, and difficult to expectorate phlegm, Rhizoma Arisaematis is commonly combined with Rhizoma Pinelliae Ternatae (*Ban Xia*).

2. Used for dizziness, vertigo, epilepsy, and spasms and contractures due to wind phlegm, Rhizoma Arisaematis can be combined with Rhizoma Gastrodiae Elatae (*Tian Ma*).

3. Used for wind damp impediment pain, Rhizoma Arisaematis can be combined with Rhizoma Atractylodis (*Cang Zhu*).

4. Used for wind phlegm blocking the channels resulting in deviation of the mouth and eyes, hemiplegia, and tetanus, Rhizoma Arisaematis can be combined with Radix Aconiti Coreani Seu Typhonii (*Bai Fu Zi*).

In addition, externally, this medicinal can be applied for welling abscesses, swellings, and snake and insect bites.

Dosage: 3-10g. Externally, use a suitable amount.

Method of use: Decoct in water and administer internally. For external application, uncooked Rhizoma Arisaematis is ground into powder, mixed with vinegar or alcohol, and applied to the affected area.

Cautions & contraindications: Use cautiously in pregnant women.

Radix Aconiti Coreani Seu Typhonii (*Bai Fu Zi*)

Nature & flavor: Acrid, sweet, and greatly warm. Has toxins.

Channel entry: Liver and stomach

Functions: Dispels wind phlegm, stabilizes spasms and contractures, resolves toxins, scatters nodulations, and stops pain

Indications:

1. Used for wind phlegm resulting in headache and one-sided headache, Radix Aconiti Coreani Seu Typhonii is commonly combined with Radix Angelicae Dahuricae (*Bai Zhi*), Rhizoma Gastrodiae Elatae (*Tian Ma*), and Rhizoma Arisaematis (*Tian Nan Xing*).

2. Used for deviation of the mouth and eyes and hemiplegia, Radix Aconiti Coreani Seu Typhonii can be combined with Bombyx Batryticatus (*Jiang Can*) and Buthus Martensis (*Quan Xie*).

3. Used for scrofulous phlegm kernels and insect and snake bites, this medicinal may be used alone applied externally.

Dosage: 3-6g. Externally, use a suitable amount.

Method of use: Decoct in water and administer internally or mash, grind into powder and mix with alcohol or cook into a paste apply to the affected area.

Cautions & contraindications: Use cautiously in pregnant women. Also, use cautiously when administering the uncooked ingredient internally.

B. Hot phlegm clearing & transforming medicinals

Radix Platycodi Grandiflori (*Jie Geng*)

Nature & flavor: Bitter, acrid, and level, *i.e.*, neutral in temperature

Channel entry: Lungs

Functions: Diffuses the lungs and dispels phlegm, expels pus and disperses welling abscesses

Indications:

1. Used for wind heat cough, throat pain, hoarse voice, cough with phlegm which is not crisp, *i.e.*, is sticky and difficult to expectorate, Radix Platycodi Grandiflori is commonly combined with Folium Mori Albi (*Sang Ye*) and Flos Chrysanthemi Morifolii (*Ju Hua*) as in *Sang Ju Yin* (Morus & Chrysanthemum Drink). For wind cold cough with watery phlegm which is white in color, one can combined Radix Platycodi Grandiflori with Semen Pruni Armeniacae (*Xing Ren*) and Folium Perillae Frutescentis (*Zi Su Ye*) as in *Xing Su San* (Armeniaca & Perilla Powder).

2. Used for lung abscess chest pain with coughing and spitting of pus and blood and yellow, foul-odored phlegm, Radix Platycodi Grandiflori is commonly combined with Radix Glycyrrhizae (*Gan Cao*) as in *Jie Geng Tang* (Platycodon Decoction).

Dosage: 3-10g

Method of use: Decoct in water and administer internally.

Fructus Trichosanthis Kirlowii (*Gua Lou*)

Nature & flavor: Sweet and cold

Channel entry: Lungs, stomach, and large intestine

Functions: Clears heat and transforms phlegm, disinhibits the qi and loosens the chest, disperses swelling and treats welling abscesses, moistens the intestines and frees the flow of the stool

Indications:

1. Used for lung heat cough with symptoms of thick, yellow-colored phlegm, coughing and spitting not easy, chest oppression, and dry stools, Fructus Trichosanthis Kirlowii is commonly combined with Radix Scutellariae Baicalensis (*Huang Qin*) and bile-processed Rhizoma Arisaematis (*Dan Nan Xing*) as in *Qing Qi Hua Tan Wan* (Clear the Qi & Transform Phlegm Pills).

Used for chest impediment and chest pain, Fructus Trichosanthis Kirlowii is commonly combined with Bulbus Allii (*Xie Bai*), Rhizoma Pinelliae Ternatae (*Ban Xia*), and white alcohol as in *Gua Lou Xie Bai Ban Xia Tang* (Trichosanthes, Allium & Pinellia Decoction). For the treatment of phlegm heat bound in the chest with chest and rib-side glomus and fullness with pain when one presses the sides, Fructus Trichosanthis Kirlowii is commonly combined with Rhizoma Pinelliae Ternatae (*Ban Xia*) and Rhizoma Coptidis Chinensis (*Huang Lian*) as in *Xiao Xian Xiong Tang* (Minor Fallen Chest Decoction).

3. Used for breast abscess and lung abscess. During the initial stage of a breast abscess with redness, swelling, heat, and pain, Fructus Trichosanthis Kirlowii is commonly combined with Herba Taraxici Monglici Cum Radice (*Pu Gong Ying*) and Flos Lonicerae Japonicae (*Jin Yin Hua*). For lung abscess with coughing and spitting of pus and blood, mostly Fructus Trichosanthis Kirlowii is combined with Herba Houttuyniae Cordatae Cum Radice (*Yu Xing Cao*).

4. Used for intestinal dryness constipation, Fructus Trichosanthis Kirlowii is commonly combined with Semen Cannabis Sativae (*Huo Ma Ren*) and Semen Pruni (*Yu Li Ren*).

Dosage: Whole Fructus Trichosanthis Kirlowii, 12-30g; Pericarpium Trichosanthis Kirlowii (*Gua Lou Pi*), 6-12g; Semen Trichosanthis Kirlowii (*Gua Lou Ren*), 10-15g

Method of use: Decoct in water and administer internally. For Chest impediment, welling abscesses, and swelling, used whole Fructus Trichosanthis Kirlowii. To clear heat and transform phlegm, disinhibit the qi and loosen the chest, use Pericarpium

Trichosanthis Kirlowii. To moisten the intestines and free the flow of the stool, use Semen Trichosanthis Kirlowii.

Cautions & contraindications: Reverses or opposes Radix Aconiti (*Wu Tou*).

Radix Trichosanthis Kirlowii (*Tian Hua Fen*)

Nature & flavor: Sweet, slightly bitter, slightly cold

Channel entry: Lungs and stomach

Functions: Clears heat and engenders fluids, disperses swelling and expels pus

Indications:

1. Used for stomach heat damaging the lungs with symptoms of a dry cough with scanty phlegm and a red tongue with scanty fur, Radix Trichosanthis Kirlowii is commonly combined with Tuber Ophiopogonis Japonici (*Mai Men Dong*) and Radix Glehniae Littoralis (*Sha Shen*) as in *Sha Shen Mai Men Dong Tang* (Glehnia & Ophiopogon Decoction).

2. Used for wasting and thirsting condition with vexatious thirst or fluid depletion in the latter stage of a warm heat disease, Radix Trichosanthis Kirlowii is commonly combined with Rhizoma Anemarrhenae Aspheloidis (*Zhi Mu*) and Rhizoma Phragmitis Communis (*Lu Gen*).

3. Used for breast abscesses with heat, swelling, hardness, and pain, Radix Trichosanthis Kirlowii is commonly combined with Squama Manitis Pentadactylis (*Chuan Shan Jia*), Fructus Gleditschiae Chinensis (*Zao Jia*), and Flos Lonicerae Japonicae (*Jin Yin Hua*).

Dosage: 10-15g

Method of use: Decoct in water and administer internally.

Cautions & contraindications: Opposes or reverses Radix Aconiti (*Wu Tou*). Use cautiously in pregnant women.

Caulis Bambusae In Taeniis (*Zhu Ru*)

Nature & flavor: Sweet and slightly cold

Channel entry: Lungs, stomach, and gallbladder

Functions: Clears heat and transforms phlegm, eliminates vexation and stops vomiting

Indications:

1. Used for lung heat cough, Caulis Bambusae In Taeniis can be combined with Fructus Trichosanthis Kirlowii (*Gua Lou*) and Radix Scutellariae Baicalensis (*Huang Qin*).

2. Used for vexatious thirst and vomiting due to heat damaging stomach fluids, Caulis Bambusae In Taeniis can be combined with Rhizoma Phragmitis Communis (*Lu Gen*).

3. Used for vexation and agitation, insomnia, easy anger, and nausea and vomiting due to hot phlegm, Caulis Bambusae can be combined with Rhizoma Pinelliae Ternatae (*Ban Xia*) and Fructus Immaturus Citri Aurantii (*Zhi Shi*).

Dosage: 4.5-12g

Method of use: Decoct in water and administer. Typically, for dispelling phlegm, the uncooked is used. Use ginger-processed for stopping vomiting.

Cautions & contraindications: It is not appropriate to use this medicinal for nausea and vomiting due to stomach cold.

Thallus Algae (*Kun Bu*)

Nature & flavor: Salty and cold

Channel entry: Spleen, stomach, and lungs

Functions: Softens the hard and scatters nodulations, disperses phlegm, disinhibits water

Indications: Used for scrofulous phlegm kernels, testicular swelling and pain, and phlegm rheum water swelling. For the treatment of scrofulous phlegm kernels, this medicinal is commonly combined with Bulbus Fritillariae Thunbergii (*Zhe Bei Mu*), Concha Ostreae (*Mu Li*), and Herba Sargassii (*Hai Zao*).

Dosage: 6-12g

Method of use: Decoct in water and administer internally.

Herba Sargassii (*Hai Zao*)

Nature & flavor: Bitter, salty, and cold

Channel entry: Lungs, spleen, kidneys, and liver

Functions: Softens the hard and scatters nodulations, disperse phlegm, disinhibits water

Indications: Used for scrofulous phlegm kernels, Herba Sargassii is often combined with Bambyx Batryticatus (*Jiang Can*), Spica Prunellae Vulgaris (*Xia Ku Cao*), and Radix Scrophulariae Ningpoensis (*Xuan Shen*).

Dosage: 6-12g

Method of use: Decoct in water and administer internally

Cautions & contraindications: Opposes or reverses Radix Glycyrrhizae (*Gan Cao*).

Bulbus Fritillariae (*Bei Mu*)

Nature & flavor: Bulbus Fritllariae Cirrhosae (*Chuan Bei Mu*) is bitter, sweet, and slightly cold. Bulbus Fritillariae Thunbergii (*Zhe Bei Mu*) is bitter and cold.

Channel entry: Both gather in the lungs and heart.

Functions: Transforms phlegm and stops cough, clears heat and scatters nodulations

Indications:

1. Bulbus Fritllariae Cirrhosae's nature is cool and sweet. Simultaneously it has the function of moistening the lungs. Therefore, it is mostly used for lung vacuity enduring cough with scanty phlegm and dry throat. In that case, it is commonly combined with Radix Glehniae Littoralis (*Sha Shen*) and Tuber Ophiopogonis Japonici (*Mai Men Dong*). Bulbus Fritillariae Thunbergii's bitterness and coldness is relatively heavy. Its power to clear fire and scatter nodulations is comparatively strong. It is mostly used for external contraction wind heat or phlegm fire depression and binding cough. For these, Bulbus Fritillariae Thunbergii is commonly combined with Folium Mori Albi (*Sang Ye*) and Fructus Arctii Lappae (*Niu Bang Zi*).

2. Used for scrofula, sores, and welling abscesses, Bulbus Fritillariae Thunbergii is quite effective. For the treatment of scrofula, it is commonly combined with Radix Scrophulariae Ningpoensis (*Xuan Shen*) and Concha Ostreae (*Mu Li*) as in *Xiao Luo Wan*

(Disperse Scrofula Pills). For the treatment of breast abscesses, it is commonly combined with Herba Taraxici Mongolici Cum Radice (*Pu Gong Ying*) and Radix Trichosanthis Kirlowii (*Tian Hua Fen*). For the treatment of lung abscesses, it is commonly combined with Herba Houttuyniae Cordatae Cum Radice (*Yu Xing Cao*) and Semen Coicis Lachryma-jobi (*Yi Yi Ren*).

Dosage: 3-10g

Method of use: Decoct in water and administer internally.

Cautions & contraindications: Reverses or opposes Radix Aconiti (*Wu Tou*).

Radix Peucedani (*Qian Hu*)

Nature & flavor: Bitter, acrid, and slightly cold

Channel entry: Lungs and spleen

Functions: Scatters wind and clears heat, downbears the qi and transforms phlegm

Indications:

1. Used for lung heat coughing and panting with profuse, thick, yellow phlegm, chest oppression, and vexation, Radix Peucedani can be combined with Cortex Radicis Mori Albi (*Sang Bai Pi*).

2. Used for external contraction wind heat headache, fever, nasal congestion, runny nose, and cough, Radix Peucedani can be combined with Radix Platycodi Grandiflori (*Jie Geng*).

Dosage: 6-10g

Method of use: Decoct in water and administer internally.

C. Cough-stopping, panting-leveling medicinals

Semen Pruni Armeniacae (*Xing Ren*)

Nature & flavor: Bitter, acrid, and slightly warm. Has small toxins.

Channel entry: Lungs and large intestine

Functions: Stops cough and levels panting, moistens the intestines and frees the flow of the stool

Indications:

1. Used for many types of cough and qi panting. For wind heat cough, Semen Pruni Armeniacae is commonly combined with Folium Mori Albi (*Sang Ye*) and Flos Chrysanthemi Morifolii (*Ju Hua*) as in *Sang Ju Yin* (Morus & Chrysanthemum Drink). For wind cold common cold with cough and qi panting, mostly it is combined with Folium Perillae Frutescentis (*Su Ye*) as in *Xing Su San* (Armeniaca & Perilla Powder). For dry heat cough, Semen Pruni Armeniacae is commonly combined with Folium Mori Albi (*Sang Ye*) and Bulbus Fritillariae (*Bei Mu*) as in *Sang Xing Tang* (Morus & Armeniaca Decoction). For lung heat coughing and panting, mostly it is combined with Herba Ephedrae (*Ma Huang*), uncooked Gypsum Fibrosum (*Shi Gao*), and Radix Glycyrrhizae (*Gan Cao*) as in *Ma Xing Shi Gan Tang* (Ephedra, Armeniaca, Gypsum & Licorice Decoction).

2. Used for intestinal dryness constipation, Semen Pruni Armeniacae is commonly combined with Semen Cannabis Sativae (*Huo Ma Ren*) and Semen Pruni Persicae (*Tao Ren*) as in *Run Chang Wan* (Moisten the Intestines Pills).

Dosage: 6-10g

Method of use: Decoct in water and administer internally.

Cautions & contraindications: Because this medicinal has some small amount of toxins, it is not appropriate to use too large a dose when administered internally so as to avoid poisoning. It should be used cautiously in children.

Semen Lepidii Seu Descurainiae (*Ting Li Zi*)

Nature & flavor: Acrid, bitter, and greatly cold

Channel entry: Lungs and urinary bladder

Functions: Drains the lungs and levels panting, disinhibits water and disperses swelling

Indications:

1. Used for phlegm rheum blockage and stagnation with symptoms of chest fullness, cough counterflow, profuse phlegm, panting with inability to breath lying down, whole body, face, and eyes superficial edema, Semen Lepidii Seu Descurainiae is commonly combined with Fructus Zizyphi Jujubae (*Da Zao*). This is then called *Ting Li Da Zao Xie Fei Tang* (Lepidium & Red Dates Drain the Lungs Decoction).

2. Used for chest and abdominal accumulation of water and inhibited urination. If water rheum collects and is retained within the intestinal spaces, this may result in abdominal fullness and a dry mouth and tongue. In this case, Semen Lepidii Seu Descurainiae is commonly combined with Radix Stephaniae Tetrandrae (*Fang Ji*), Semen Zanthoxyli Bungeani (*Jiao Mu*), and Radix Et Rhizoma Rhei (*Da Huang*). This is called *Ji Jiao Li Huang Wan* (Stephania, Zanthoxylum, Lepidium & Rhubarb Pills). If there is chest and rib-side accumulation of water with dry, bound stools and short, scanty urination, Semen Lepidii Seu Descurainiae is commonly combined with Semen Pruni Armeniacae (*Xing Ren*) and Radix Et Rhizoma Rhei (*Da Huang*) as in *Da Xian Xiong Wan* (Major Fallen Chest Pills).

Dosage: 3-10g

Method of use: Decoct in water and administer internally.

Cautions & contraindications: This medicinal is contraindicated in case of lung vacuity panting and cough and spleen vacuity swelling and fullness.

Fructus Perillae Frutescentis (*Zi Su Zi*)

Nature & flavor: Acrid and warm

Channel entry: Lungs and large intestine

Functions: Stops cough and levels panting, downbears the qi and disperses phlegm, moistens the intestines and frees the flow of the stool

Indications:

1. Used for phlegm blockage and qi counterflow with cough and qi panting, Fructus Perillae Frutescentis is commonly combined with Semen Sinapis Albae (*Bai Jie Zi*) and Semen Raphani Sativi (*Lai Fu Zi*). This is then called *San Zi Yang Qin Tang* (Three Seeds Nourish the Aged Decoction).

2. Used for phlegm drool blockage and exuberance with chest and diaphragmatic fullness and oppression, cough, panting respiration, and shortness of breath categorized as repletion above and vacuity below, Fructus Perillae Frutescentis is commonly combined with Cortex Magnoliae Officinalis (*Hou Po*) and Pericarpium Citri Reticulatae (*Chen Pi*) as in *Su Zi Jiang Qi Tang* (Perilla Seed Downbear the Qi Decoction).

3. Used for intestinal dryness constipation, Fructus Perillae Frutescentis is commonly combined with Semen Cannabis Sativae (*Huo Ma Ren*) and Semen Pruni Armeniacae (*Xing Ren*).

Dosage: 6-10g

Method of use: Decoct in water and administer internally.

Cautions & contraindications: This medicinal is contraindicated if there is spleen vacuity loose stools.

Radix Asteris Tatarici (*Zi Wan*)

Nature & flavor: Acrid, bitter, and slightly warm

Channel entry: Lungs

Functions: Moistens the lungs and descends the qi, disperses phlegm and stops coughing

Indications: Used for various types of coughing and panting. For coughing and panting with profuse phlegm and counterflow qi, Radix Asteris Tatarici can be combined with Flos Tussilaginis Farfarae (*Kuan Dong Hua*). For acute or chronic hacking of blood, Radix Asteris Tatarici can be combined with Radix Stemonae (*Bai Bu*). For chronic dry cough due to heat damaging the fluids, Radix Asteris Tatarici can be combined with Tuber Ophiopogonis Japonici (*Mai Men Dong*), Radix Scutellariae Baicalensis (*Huang Qin*), and Cortex Radicis Mori Albi (*Sang Bai Pi*). For cough with profuse phlegm, panting and wheezing, and spontaneous perspiration, Radix Asteris Tatarici can be combined with Fructus Schisandrae Chinensis (*Wu Wei Zi*).

Dosage: 4.5-10g

Method of use: Decoct in water and administer internally. For external contraction cough, it is appropriate to use uncooked. Honey mix-fried is more effective for moistening the lungs and for cases of enduring cough due to lung vacuity.

Flos Tussilaginis Farfarae (*Kuan Dong Hua*)

Nature & flavor: Acrid, slightly bitter, and warm

Channel entry: Lungs

Functions: Moistens the lungs and descends the qi, stops coughing and transforms phlegm

Indications: Used for various new and enduring coughs and panting. For the treatment of coughing and panting due to phlegm obstructing the lungs, Flos Tussilaginis Farfarae can be combined with Semen Pruni Armeniacae (*Xing Ren*). For dry cough due to lung yin vacuity, it can be combined with Bulbus Lilii (*Bai He*).

Dosage: 4.5-10g

Method of use: Decoct in water and administer internally. For external contraction cough, use uncooked. For enduring cough due to vacuity, use mix-fried.

Cautions & contraindications: Due to this medicinal's warm nature, it should be used cautiously in heat coughs.

Folium Eriobotryae Japonicae (*Pi Pa Ye*)

Nature & flavor: Bitter and slightly cold

Channel entry: Lungs and stomach

Functions: Clears the lungs and stops coughing, downbears counterflow and stops vomiting

Indications:

1. Used for lung heat cough, Folium Eriobotryae Japonicae is commonly combined with Semen Pruni Armeniacae (*Xing Ren*).

2. Used for vomiting and spitting. For the treatment of vexatious thirst and vomiting due to damaged fluids in the latter stage of a warm heat disease, Folium Eriobotryae Japonicae can be combined with Rhizoma Phragmitis Communis (*Lu Gen*). For spitting of blood due to damage to the network vessels by heat evils, Folium Eriobotryae Japonicae can be combined with Rhizoma Imperatae Cylindricae (*Bai Mao Gen*). And for liver-stomach depressive heat vomiting, Folium Eriobotryae Japonicae can be combined with Radix Scutellariae Baicalensis (*Huang Qin*) and Rhizoma Cyperi Rotundi (*Xiang Fu*).

Dosage: 6-12g

Method of use: Decoct in water and administer internally. For stopping coughing, use mix-fried. For stopping vomiting, use uncooked.

Cautions & contraindications: This medicinal is contraindicated in vomiting due to stomach cold and cough due to external contraction of wind cold.

Radix Stemonae (*Bai Bu*)

Nature & flavor: Sweet, bitter, and slightly warm

Channel entry: Lungs

Functions: Moistens the lungs, descends the qi, and stops coughing, kills worms

Indications:

1. Used for acute and chronic coughs of various types. However, Radix Stemonae is most effective for chronic coughs due to lung yin vacuity dryness, in which case, it can be combined with uncooked Rehmanniae (*Sheng Di*), Tuber Ophiopogonis Japonici (*Mai Men Dong*), Bulbus Fritillariae Cirrhosae (*Chuan Bei Mu*), and Gelatinum Corii Asini (*E Jiao*) as in *Yue Hua Wan* (Moon Luster Pills).

2. Used both internally and externally for various types of worms. For head and body lice or fleas, Radix Stemonae can be applied externally as either a tincture or wash. For pinworms, it make be taken internally as a retention enema.

Dosage: 6-10g. Externally, use a suitable amount.

Method of use: Decoct in water and administer internally or use as a wash externally or soak in alcohol and use as a tincture applied to the affected area. Honey mix-fried Radix Stemonae is more effective for moistening the lungs and stopping cough.

Cautions & contraindications: This medicinal is contraindicated in case of spleen vacuity loose stools.

Cortex Radicis Mori Albi (*Sang Bai Pi*)

Nature & flavor: Bitter and cold

Channel entry: Lungs, liver, and spleen

Functions: Drains the lungs and levels panting, moves water and disperses swelling

Indications:

1. Used for coughing and panting. For the treatment of lung heat coughing and panting with fever, thick phlegm, fever, and vexatious thirst, Cortex Radicis Mori Albi can be combined with Cortex Radicis Lycii Chinensis (*Di Gu Pi*). For the treatment of wind cold cough in a person with enduring phlegm deep-lying in the lungs, Cortex Radicis Mori Albi is commonly combined with Herba Ephedrae (*Ma Huang*), Semen Pruni Armeniacae (*Xing Ren*), and Fructus Perillae Frutescentis (*Zi Su Zi*) as in *Hua Gai San* (Florid Canopy Powder).

2. Used for superficial edema and inhibited urination, Cortex Radicis Mori Albi can be combined with Pericarpium Arecae Catechu (*Da Fu Pi*).

Dosage: 6-12g

Method of use: Decoct in water and administer internally. For moving water, use uncooked. For leveling panting and stopping cough, use mix-fried.

Cautions & contraindications: This medicinal is not appropriate for use in lung cold cough and wind cold cough.

4

Draining & precipitating medicinals

Medicinals which are capable of draining the abdomen or glossing and disinhibiting the large intestine in order to promote the expulsion of the stools are called draining and precipitating medicinals. Such medicinals have the effect of freeing the flow of and disinhibiting the stool, clearing heat and draining fire, expelling water and dispersing swelling and are suitable for use in constipation, intestinal tract accumulation and stagnation, replete heat internally binding, and water swelling and collecting of rheum interior repletion conditions.

Draining and precipitating medicinals can be subdivided into the three types of attacking and precipitating, moistening and precipitating, and drastically precipitating expelling water medicinals. Because attacking and precipitating and drastically precipitating medicinals are very strong and harsh, they get their effects very quickly but also easily damage the righteous qi. Moistening and precipitating medicinals are moderate and harmonious and do not damage the righteous qi.

When using draining and precipitating medicinals, one should pay attention to the following points: If there is interior repletion with a simultaneous exterior pattern, one should first resolve the exterior and then attack the interior or, if necessary, resolve both the exterior and interior at the same time. If there is an interior repletion with righteous vacuity, it is essential to attack and supplement simultaneously. Because this category of medicinals easily damages the stomach qi, as soon as they get their effect, they should be stopped and overdosage should be avoided.

A. Attacking & precipitating medicinals

Radix Et Rhizoma Rhei (*Da Huang*)

Nature & flavor: Bitter and cold

Channel entry: Spleen, stomach, large intestine, liver, and heart

Functions: Drains heat and frees the flow of the stool, cools the blood and resolves toxins, quickens the blood and dispels stasis

Indications:

1. Used for intestinal tract accumulation and heat (or of heat) with constipated, bound stools. This ingredient is a main medicinal for the treatment of accumulation and stagnation constipation. Due to its bitter, cold nature and flavor, it is especially suitable for heat binding constipation. For stomach and intestine replete heat constipation with abdominal pain which refuses pressure, Radix Et Rhizoma Rhei is commonly combined with Mirabilitum (*Mang Xiao*), Fructus Immaturus Citri Aurantii (*Zhi Shi*), and Cortex Magnoliae Officinalis (*Hou Po*) as in *Da* and *Xiao Cheng Qi Tang* (Major and Minor Order the Qi Decoctions). For heat binding damaging yin with non-freely flowing stools, Radix Et Rhizoma Rhei can be combined with uncooked Radix Rehmanniae (*Sheng Di*) and Radix Scrophulariae Ningpoensis (*Xuan Shen*) as in *Zeng Ye Cheng Qi Tang* (Increase Humors Order the Qi Decoction). If there is spleen yang insufficiency with chill accumulation constipation, one can also combine Radix Et Rhizoma Rhei with Radix Codonopsitis Pilosulae (*Dang Shen*) and Radix Lateralis Praeparatus Aconiti Carmichaeli (*Fu Zi*) as in *Wen Pi Tang* (Warm the Spleen Decoction).

In addition, this ingredient can be used for intestinal tract damp heat downward dysentery with loose stools which are not crisp, *i.e.*, which are sticky and hard to evacuate. In that case, Radix Et Rhizoma Rhei is mostly combined with Radix Paeoniae Lactiflorae (*Shao Yao*), Radix Scutellariae Baicalensis (*Huang Qin*), and Radix Auklandiae Lappae (*Mu Xiang*) as in *Shao Yao Tang* (Peony Decoction).

2. Used for blood heat frenetic movement spitting of blood and spontaneous ejection of blood as well as fire evils flaring upward red eyes, sore throat, and gum swelling and pain, Radix Et Rhizoma Rhei is commonly combined with Rhizoma Coptidis Chinensis (*Huang Lian*), Radix Scutellariae Baicalensis (*Huang Qin*), and Calculus Bovis (*Niu Huang*) as in *Xie Xin Tang* (Drain the Heart Decoction) and *Niu Huang Jie Du Wan* (Bezoar Resolve Toxins Pills).

3. Used for heat toxin sores and welling abscesses as well as burns. In the treatment of the initial stage of upper back welling abcesses, Radix Et Rhizoma Rhei is commonly combined with Radix Angelicae Dahuricae (*Bai Zhi*) as in *Shuang Jie Gui Jin Wan* (Dual Resolving Precious [as] Gold Pills). For the treatment of intestinal abscess with abdominal pain, Radix Et Rhizoma Rhei can be combined with Cortex Radicis Moutan (*Dan Pi*) and Mirabilitum (*Mang Xiao*) as in *Da Huang Mu Dan Tang* (Rhubarb & Moutan Decoction). For the treatment of scalds and burns, it can be combined with Radix Sanguisorbae (*Di Yu*). Equal amounts of each are powdered and mixed with roasted sesame oil and applied to the affected area.

4. Used for postpartum static blood abdominal pain, concretions and conglomerations, accumulations and gatherings, and injury due to fall and strike resulting in amassment of blood. For the treatment of postpartum static pain below the navel and lower abdominal

cramping and pain refusing pressure, Radix Et Rhizoma Rhei is commonly combined with Semen Pruni Persicae (*Tao Ren*) and Eupolyphaga Seu Opisthoplatia (*Zhe Chong*) as in *Xia Yu Xue Tang* (Precipitate Static Blood Decoction). For liver-spleen blood stasis with enlarged abdomen and blue-green sinews, *i.e.*, veins, one can combine Radix Et Rhizoma Rhei with Rhizoma Curcumae Zedoariae (*E Zhu*) and Radix Ligustici Wallichii (*Chuan Xiong*) as in *Tiao Gong Yin* (Regulate the Palace Drink). For static blood amassing under the ribs due to detriment and damage from fall and strike accompanied by unbearable pain, Radix Et Rhizoma Rhei is commonly combined with Radix Angelicae Sinensis (*Dang Gui*) and Flos Carthami Tinctorii (*Hong Hua*) as in *Fu Yuan Huo Xue Tang* (Recover the Source & Quicken the Blood Decoction). For heat falling into the lower burning with qi and blood obstruction and stagnation accompanied by lower abdominal hardness and fullness, mania, but uninhibited urination, Radix Et Rhizoma Rhei is commonly combined with Hirudo (*Shui Zhi*) and Semen Pruni Persicae (*Tao Ren*) as in *Di Dang Tang* (Dead-on Decoction) and *Tao Ren Cheng Qi Tang* (Persica Order the Qi Decoction).

In addition, because this ingredient has the function of clearing and discharging dampness and heat, disinhibiting the gallbladder and receding jaundice, it can also be used for jaundice and strangury. For the treatment of jaundice, Radix Et Rhizoma Rhei is commonly combined with Herba Artemisiae Capillaris (*Yin Chen Hao*) and Fructus Gardeniae Jasminoidis (*Zhi Zi*) as in *Yin Chen Hao Tang* (Capillaris Decoction). For the treatment of urinary strangury, dribbling, astringency, and pain, Radix Et Rhizoma Rhei is commonly combined with Caulis Akebiae (*Mu Tong*) and Semen Plantaginis (*Che Qian Zi*) as in *Ba Zheng San* (Eight [Ingredients] Correcting Powder).

Dosage: 3-15g. Externally, use a suitable amount.

Method of use: Decoct in water and administer internally. When used for the treatment of draining and precipitating, it should be added later or washed down as a powder with water. The power of the uncooked is drastic, while the power of the cooked is milder. For quickening the blood and transforming stasis, one should use alcohol-processed. For stopping bleeding, one should used stir-fried till carbonized.

Cautions & contraindications: This medicinal should be used cautiously or is contraindicated in pregnant women, women having their menses, or lactating women.

Mirabilitum (*Mang Xiao*)

Nature & flavor: Salty, bitter, and cold

Channel entry: Stomach and large intestine

Functions: Drains and precipitates, softens the hard, clears heat and resolves toxins

Indications:

1. Used for intestinal and stomach replete heat accumulation and stagnation with dry, bound stools, Mirabilitum is commonly combined with Radix Et Rhizoma Rhei (*Da Huang*) as in *Da Cheng Qi Tang* (Major Order the Qi Decoction) and *Tiao Wei Cheng Qi Tang* (Regulate the Stomach & Order the Qi Decoction).

2. Used for throat pain, oral sores, and red eyes. This ingredient when used externally is able to clear heat and resolve toxins. In the treatment of throat pain and oral sores, Mirabilitum is commonly combined with Borax (*Peng Sha*) and Borneol (*Bing Pian*) as in *Bing Peng San* (Borneol & Borax Powder). For the treatment of red, swollen, painful eyes, a suitable amount of refined Mirabilitum (*Xuan Ming Fen*) is spread on a piece of tofu and seamed. The resulting liquid is used as drops for the eyes.

In addition, this ingredient can be used to treat breast abscess swelling and pain when applied externally. It can also be used to return the milk, *i.e.*, terminate lactation.

Dosage: 3-15g. Externally, use a suitable amount.

Method of use: Dissolve in the herbal juice after decoction or dissolve in boiling water and take.

Cautions & contraindications: Contraindicated in pregnant women.

B. Moistening & precipitating medicinals

Semen Cannabis Sativae (*Huo Ma Ren*)

Nature & flavor: Sweet and level

Channel entry: Spleen, stomach, and large intestine

Functions: Moistens the intestines and frees the flow of the stool

Indications: Used for fluid debility and blood vacuity constipation in the elderly, postpartum women, and those with bodily vacuity, Semen Cannabis Sativae is commonly combined with Radix Angelicae Sinensis (*Dang Gui*) and cooked Radix Rehmanniae (*Shu Di*) as in *Yi Xue Run Chang Wan* (Boost the Blood & Moisten the Intestines Pills). For heat evils damaging yin or habitual bodily fire effulgence with constipated, bound stools and hemorrhoids or recalcitrant constipation, it can be combined with Radix Et Rhizoma

Rhei (*Da Huang*) and Fructus Immaturus Citri Aurantii (*Zhi Shi*) as in *Ma Zi Ren Wan* (Cannabis Seed Pills).

Dosage: 10-30g

Method of use: Decoct in water and administer internally.

Cautions & contraindications: One should not use too large a dose. If 60-120g are administered internally at one time, this can cause poisoning with vomiting and diarrhea, numbness of the four extremities, and, in severe cases, unconsciousness.

Semen Pruni (*Yu Li Ren*)

Nature & flavor: Acrid, bitter, and level

Channel entry: Large intestine, small intestine, and spleen

Functions: Moistens the intestines and frees the flow of the stool, disinhibits water and disperses swelling

Indications:

1. Used for fluid withering intestinal dryness constipation, Semen Pruni is commonly combined with Semen Pruni Armeniacae (*Xing Ren*) and Semen Biotae Orientalis (*Bai Zi Ren*) as in *Wu Ren Wan* (Five Seeds Pills).

2. Used for water swelling abdominal fullness, leg qi superficial edema, and inhibited urination, Semen Pruni is commonly combined with Cortex Radicis Mori Albi (*Sang Bai Pi*) and Semen Phaseoli Calcarati (*Chi Xiao Dou*) as in *Yu Li Ren Tang* (Prune Pit Decoction).

Dosage: 6-12g

Method of use: Decoct in water and administer internally.

Cautions & contraindications: Use cautiously in pregnant women.

C. Drastic precipitating & expelling water medicinals

Radix Euphorbiae Kansui (*Gan Sui*)

Nature & flavor: Bitter and cold. Has small toxins.

Channel entry: Lungs, kidneys, and large intestine

Functions: Drains water and expels rheum, disperses swelling and scatters nodulations

Indications:

1. Used for bodily and facial superficial edema, upper abdominal water swelling, and chest and rib-side accumulation of fluids. Because this ingredient is such a drastic draining water and expelling rheum medicinal, after administering it, there can be severe diarrhea. For the treatment of water swelling abdominal fullness, Radix Euphorbiae Kansui is commonly combined with Semen Pharbiditis (*Qian Niu Zi*) as in *Er Qi Tang* (Two Qi Decoction). For the treatment of chest and abdominal water rheum collecting internally, phlegm rheum accumulation and gathering, chest and rib-side drawing pain, and cough counterflow, panting, and fullness, Radix Euphorbiae Kansui is commonly combined with Fructus Zizyphi Jujubae (*Da Zao*), Radix Euphorbiae Seu Knoxiae (*Da Ji*), and Flos Daphnes Genkwae (*Yuan Hua*) as in *Shi Zao Tang* (Ten Dates Decoction). For water rheum and heat evils binding in the chest, Radix Euphorbiae Kansui can be combined with Radix Et Rhizoma Rhei (*Da Huang*) and Mirabilitum (*Mang Xiao*). This is called *Da Xian Xiong Tang* (Major Fallen Chest Decoction).

In modern times, Radix Euphorbiae Kansui is commonly combined with Radix Et Rhizoma Rhei (*Da Huang*) and Cortex Magnoliae Officinalis (*Hou Po*) as in *Gan Sui Tong Jie Tang* (Euphorbia Free the Flow of Binding Decoction) for the treatment of heavy pattern intestinal obstruction and intestinal cavity accumulation of fluids.

2. Used for welling abscesses, swelling, sores, and toxins, Radix Euphorbiae Kansui is ground into powder, mixed with water, and applied externally.

In addition, Radix Euphorbiae Kansui can also be used for wind phlegm epilepsy due to its ability to expel phlegm. In that case, it is ground into powder, placed inside a pig's heart, and roasted excessively. This is then powdered, mixed with Cinnabar (*Zhu Sha*), made into pills, and administered.

Dosage: 0.5-1.5g. Externally, use a suitable amount of uncooked.

Method of use: It should be taken as pills or powders. It should not be decocted.

Cautions & contraindications: This medicinal is contraindicated in pregnant women and those with bodily vacuity. It opposes or reverses Radix Glycyrrhizae (*Gan Cao*).

Radix Euphorbiae Seu Knoxiae (*Da Ji*)

Nature & flavor: Bitter and cold. Has toxins.

Channel entry: Lungs, kidneys, and large intestine

Functions: Drains water and expels rheum, disperses swelling and scatters nodulations

Indications:

1. Used for bodily and facial superficial edema, upper abdominal water swelling, and chest and rib-side accumulation of fluids. Because Radix Euphorbiae Seu Knoxiae is similar in action to Radix Euphorbiae Kansui (*Gan Sui*), but its power is somewhat less drastic, it is commonly combined with Radix Euphorbiae Kansui and Flos Daphnes Genkwae (*Yuan Hua*) as in *Shi Zao Tang* (Ten Dates Decoction) and *Zhou Ju Wan* (Boat & Cart Pills).

2. Used for heat toxin welling abcesses, swelling, sores, and toxins as well as phlegm fire coagulation and gathering scrofulous phlegm kernels, Radix Euphorbiae Seu Knoxiae can be both administered internally and applied externally.

Dosage: 0.5-1.5g

Method of use: Mostly this medicinal is taken in pills and powders.

Cautions & contraindications: This medicinal is contraindicated in pregnant women and those with bodily vacuity. It opposes or reverses Radix Glycyrrhizae (*Gan Cao*).

Flos Daphnes Genkwae (*Yuan Hua*)

Nature & flavor: Acrid, bitter, and warm. Has toxins.

Channel entry: Lungs, kidneys, and large intestine

Functions: Drains water and expels rheum, dispels phlegm and stops cough. Used externally, kills worms and treats sores.

Indications:

1. Used for bodily and facial superficial edema, upper abdominal water swelling, and chest and rib-side accumulation of fluids. Because this medicinal's water-draining action is the same as that of Radix Euphrobiae Kansui (*Gan Sui*) and Radix Euphorbiae Seu Knoxiae (*Da Ji*), it is commonly combined with those two medicinals as in *Shi Zao Tang* (Ten Dates Decoction) and *Zhou Ju Wan* (Boat & Cart Pills).

2. Used for profuse phlegm cough, the combination of Flos Daphnes Genkwae and Fructus Zizyphi Jujubae (*Da Zao*) is effective in the treatment of cold damp pattern chronic bronchitis.

3. Used for head sores, bald white scalp sores, and stubborn lichen, Flos Daphnes Genkwae can either be used alone ground into powder or mixed with Realgar (*Xiong Huang*) and pig fat, mixed into an ointment, and applied externally.

Dosage: 1.5-3g

Method of use: This medicinal is mostly taken in pills and powders. Externally, use a suitable amount.

Cautions & contraindications: This medicinal is contraindicated in pregnant women and those with bodily vacuity. It opposes or reverses Radix Glycyrrhizae (*Gan Cao*).

5

Dampness-dispelling medicinals

Medicinals whose effects are mainly to dispel and eliminate wind dampness and resolve and eliminate impediment pain are called wind damp dispelling medicinals. Those whose qi and flavor are penetrating and aromatic and which have the actions of fortifying the spleen and transforming dampness are called penetrating, aromatic, dampness-transforming medicinals. And those which are able to free the flow of and disinhibit the water passageways, seep and discharge water dampness are called water-disinhibiting, dampness-seeping medicinals. Since dispelling dampness, transforming dampness, and seeping dampness all disperse and eliminate damp evils internally in the body, as a group they are, therefore, called dampness-dispelling medicinals.

This group of medicinals is suitable for use in wind cold damp impediment, water swelling, strangury disease, jaundice, bound stones, dampness obstructing the middle burner, and spleen movement loss of constancy, *i.e.*, normalcy, conditions. Because of their warm, dry natures and their power to disinhibit water, they can easily consume and damage yin and blood. Therefore, they should be used cautiously in case of yin debility, blood vacuity, and fluid damage.

A. Wind damp dispelling medicinals

Radix Angelicae Pubescentis (*Du Huo*)

Nature & flavor: Acrid, bitter, and slightly warm

Channel entry: Kidneys and urinary bladder

Functions: Dispels wind, overcomes dampness, and stops pain, scatters cold and resolves the exterior

Indications:

1. Used for wind dampness impediment pain, Radix Angelicae Pubescentis is especially appropriate for impediment conditions of the lower half of the body. Therefore, this medicinal is a first choice for low back and leg aching and pain and wilting and impediment of the two feet inability to walk or stand. For these purposes, it is commonly combined with Ramulus Loranthi Seu Visci (*Sang Ji Sheng*), Radix Gentianae

Macrophyllae (*Qin Jiao*), and Radix Achyranthis Bidentatae (*Niu Xi*) as in *Du Huo Ji Sheng Tang* (Angelica Pubescens & Loranthus Decoction).

2. Used for external contraction wind cold with internal cold evils conditions with symptoms of headache, whole body joint heaviness, soreness, and pain, and slight aversion to wind and cold, Radix Angelicae Pubescentis is commonly combined with Radix Gentianae Macrophyllae (*Qin Jiao*) as in *Du Huo Sheng Shi Tang* (Angelica Pubescens Overcome Dampness Decoction).

Dosage: 3-10g

Method of use: Decoct in water and administer internally.

Radix Stephaniae Tetrandrae (*Fang Ji*)

Nature & flavor: Bitter, acrid, and cold

Channel entry: Urinary bladder, kidneys, and spleen

Functions: Dispels wind and stops pain, disinhibits water and disperses swelling

Indications:

1. Used for wind cold impediment pain. For the treatment of wind cold natured joint aching and pain, Radix Stephaniae Tetrandrae is commonly combined with Rhizoma Atractylodis Macrocephalae (*Bai Zhu*) and Cortex Cinnamomi Cassiae (*Rou Gui*) as in *Fang Ji Tang* (Stephania Decoction). For the treatment of damp heat obstructing and stagnating in the channels and network vessels with joint aching and pain or leg qi swelling and pain, Radix Stephaniae Tetrandrae can be combined with Radix Achyranthis Bidentatae (*Niu Xi*) and Cortex Phellodendri (*Huang Bai*).

2. Used for lower burner damp heat, water swelling, abdominal water, and inhibited urination. For the treatment of generalized water swelling with a floating pulse, a heavy body, sweating, and aversion to wind, Radix Stephaniae Tetrandrae is commonly combined with Radix Astragali Membranacei (*Huang Qi*) and Rhizoma Atractylodis Macrocephalae (*Bai Zhu*) as in *Fang Ji Huang Qi Tang* (Stephania & Astragalus Decoction). For superficial edema of the four limbs and inhibited urination skin water, Radix Stephaniae Tetrandrae can be combined with Sclerotium Poriae Cocos (*Fu Ling*) and Radix Astragali Membranacei (*Huang Qi*) as in *Fang Ji Fu Ling Tang* (Stephania & Poria Decoction). For phlegm rheum conditions with water qi in the intestinal spaces, abdominal region distention and fullness, and a dry mouth and tongue, it can be combined

with Semen Zanthoxyli Bungeani (*Jiao Mu*), Semen Lepidii Tinglii (*Ting Li Zi*) and Radix Et Rhizoma Rhei (*Da Huang*) ground into powder and made into pills. This is called *Ji Jiao Li Huang Wan* (Stephania, Zanthoxylum, Lepidium & Rhubarb Pills).

Dosage: 3-10g

Method of use: Decoct in water and administer internally. For the disinhibiting of water and dispersion of swelling, one should use Radix Stephaniae Tetrandrae (*Han Fang Ji*). For dispelling wind, eliminating dampness, and stopping pain, one should use Radix Aristolochiae Seu Cocculi (*Guang Fang Ji*).

Cautions & contraindications: Because this medicinal's bitter coldness is relatively severe, it easily damages the stomach qi. Therefore, it is contraindicated in those with bodily weakness and yin vacuity as well as devitalized eating and drinking.

Radix Clematidis Chinensis (*Wei Ling Xian*)

Nature & flavor: Acrid, salty, and warm

Channel entry: Urinary bladder

Functions: Dispels wind and eliminates dampness, frees the flow of the network vessels and stops pain

Indications: Used for wind damp impediment, numbness of the extremities, sinew vessel spasms and contractures, and inhibited bending and extending. For joint and sinew aching and pain especially in the upper body, Radix Clematidis Chinensis is commonly combined with Radix Et Rhizoma Notopterygii (*Qiang Huo*). For joint and sinew aching and pain especially in the lower extremities, this medicinal is commonly combined with Radix Achyranthis Bidentatae (*Niu Xi*).

In addition, this medicinal can also be used to treat fish bones stuck in the throat.

Dosage: 6-10g

Method of use: Decoct in water and administer internally. For fish bones stuck in the throat, take with vinegar and brown sugar.

Cautions & contraindications: This medicinal is contraindicated in qi and blood dual vacuity patterns.

Fructus Chaenomelis Lagenariae (*Mu Gua*)

Nature & flavor: Sour and warm

Channel entry: Liver and spleen

Functions: Levels the liver and soothes the sinews, harmonizes the stomach and transforms dampness

Indications:

1. Used for damp impediment pain, low back and knee soreness, heaviness, aching, and pain, Fructus Chaenomelis Lagenariae is commonly combined with Radix Angelicae Pubescentis (*Du Huo*).

2. Used for summerheat dampness vomiting and diarrhea with possible spasms and contractures of the calf muscles, Fructus Chaenomelis Lagenariae can be combined with Herba Agastachis Seu Pogostemi (*Huo Xiang*) and Fructus Amomi (*Sha Ren*).

3. Used for spasms and contractures of the sinews and vessels due to blood vacuity, Fructus Chaenomelis Lagenariae can be combined with Radix Angelicae Sinensis (*Dang Gui*) and Radix Albus Paeoniae Lactiflorae (*Bai Shao*).

Dosage: 6-10g

Method of use: Decoct in water and administer internally.

Cautions & contraindications: This medicinal is contraindicated in exterior patterns.

Fructus Xanthii Sibirici (*Cang Er Zi*)

Nature & flavor: Acrid, bitter, and warm. Has toxins.

Channel entry: Lungs and liver

Functions: Scatters wind dampness, frees the flow of the orifice of the nose

Indications:

1. Used for wind cold headache, runny nose, and deep source nasal congestion, Fructus Xanthii Sibirici is commonly combined with Flos Magnoliae Liliflorae (*Xin Yi Hua*). For the treatment of acute wind heat patterns, one can also add Gypsum Fibrosum (*Shi Gao*)

and Radix Scutellariae Baicalensis (*Huang Qin*). For chronic wind heat patterns with blood stasis and brewing toxins, one can add Radix Rubrus Paeoniae Lactiflorae (*Chi Shao*) and Flos Lonicerae Japonicae (*Jin Yin Hua*). And for allergic rhinitis with clear, watery nasal phlegm which dribbles and drips without cease, one can add Fructus Schisandrae Chinensis (*Wu Wei Zi*) and Fructus Rosae Laevigatae (*Jin Ying Zi*).

2. Used for wind damp impediment pain, spasms and contractures, and numbness, Fructus Xanthii Sibirici can be combined with Radix Clematidis Chinensis (*Wei Ling Xian*).

3. Used for wind rash itching, Fructus Xanthii Sibirici can be combined with Fructus Tribuli Terrestris (*Bai Ji Li*) and administered internally or used as a fumigation and wash externally.

Dosage: 3-10g. Externally, use a suitable amount.

Method of use: Decoct in water and administer internally or use the decoction as an external fumigation and wash.

Ramulus Mori Albi (*Sang Zhi*)

Nature & flavor: Bitter and level

Channel entry: Liver

Functions: Dispels wind dampness, disinhibits the joints and sinews

Indications: Used for wind damp impediment pain, soreness, and numbness, Ramulus Mori Albi can be combined with Radix Clematidis Chinensis (*Wei Ling Xian*).

Dosage: 10-15g

Method of use: Decoct in water and administer internally.

Cortex Radicis Acanthopanacis (*Wu Jia Pi*)

Nature & flavor: Acrid, bitter, and warm

Channel entry: Liver and kidneys

Functions: Dispels wind dampness, supplements the liver and kidneys, strengthens the sinews and bones

Indications:

1. Used for wind damp impediment pain and spasm and contracture of the sinew vessels, Cortex Radicis Acanthopanacis can be combined with Radix Clematidis Chinensis (*Wei Ling Xian*), Radix Et Rhizoma Notopterygii (*Qiang Huo*), and Radix Gentianae Macrophyllae (*Qin Jiao*).

2. Used for liver-kidney vacuity sinew and bone wilting and flaccidity, children's slow walking, and lack of strength, Cortex Radicis Acanthopanacis can be combined with Ramulus Loranthi Seu Visci (*Sang Ji Sheng*) and Radix Dipsaci (*Xu Duan*).

In addition, this medicinal has an effect of disinhibiting water and dispersing swelling. Therefore, it can be used for water swelling.

Dosage: 6-10g

Method of use: Decoct in water and administer internally.

Ramulus Loranthi Seu Visci (*Sang Ji Sheng*)

Nature & flavor: Bitter, sweet, and level

Channel entry: Liver and kidneys

Functions: Dispels wind dampness, supplements the liver and kidneys, strengthens the sinews and bones, and nourishes the blood and quiets the fetus

Indications:

1. Used for wind damp impediment pain, low back and knee soreness and pain. This ingredient is able to both dispel wind dampness and supplement the liver and kidneys and strengthen the sinews and bones. Therefore, it is especially suitable if there is both liver-kidney insufficiency as well as inhibited sinews and bones with low back and knee soreness and pain. In that case, Ramulus Loranthi Seu Visci is commonly combined with Radix Angelicae Pubescentis (*Du Huo*) and Radix Achyranthis Bidentatae (*Niu Xi*) as in *Du Huo Ji Sheng Tang* (Angelica Pubescens & Loranthus Decoction).

2. Used for blood vacuity fetal stirring restlessness and fetal leakage precipitation of blood, Ramulus Loranthi Seu Visci is commonly combined with Radix Angelicae Sinensis (*Dang Gui*), Gelatinum Corii Asini (*E Jiao*), and Radix Dipsaci (*Xu Duan*) as in *Sang Ji Sheng San* (Loranthus Powder).

In addition, this medicinal can be used for high blood pressure disease.

Dosage: 10-30g. It may also be used in larger doses up to 60g.

Method of use: Decoct in water and administer internally.

B. Penetrating, aromatic, dampness-transforming medicinals

Rhizoma Atractylodis (*Cang Zhu*)

Nature & flavor: Acrid, bitter, and warm

Channel entry: Spleen and stomach

Functions: Dries dampness and fortifies the spleen, dispels wind and overcomes dampness, eliminates visual obstruction and brightens the eyes

Indications:

1. Used for dampness obstructing the middle burner with symptoms of stomach duct and abdominal distention and fullness, devitalized eating and drinking, nausea and vomiting, fatigue, lack of strength, and a turbid, slimy tongue coating. This is a main medicinal for drying dampness and fortifying the spleen. In that case, Rhizoma Atractylodis is commonly combined with Cortex Magnoliae Officinalis (*Hou Po*) and Pericarpium Citri Reticulatae (*Chen Pi*) as in *Ping Wei San* (Level the Stomach Powder).

2. Used for wind cold damp impediment with joint and limb aching and pain, Rhizoma Atractylodis is commonly combined with Radix Et Rhizoma Notopterygii (*Qiang Huo*) and Ramulus Cinnamomi Cassiae (*Gui Zhi*). Because this medicinal has the ability to dispel wind and overcome dampness at the same time as effusing sweat, it can also be used for external contraction exterior pattern headache with no sweating and limb soreness and pain. In that case, it is commonly combined with Radix Et Rhizoma Notopterygii (*Qiang Huo*) and Radix Ledebouriellae Divaricatae (*Fang Feng*). For the treatment of damp heat pouring downward with foot and knee swelling and pain, it is commonly combined with Cortex Phellodendri (*Huang Bai*) and Radix Achyranthis Bidentatae (*Niu Xi*) as in *San Miao San* (Three Wonders Powder).

3. Used for eyes diseases such as internal and external visual obstructions, clear-eyed blindness, and night blindness. For these purposes, Rhizoma Atractylodis may be used alone or together with Semen Sesami Indici (*Hei Zhi Ma*) and pig liver as in *Cang Zhu Wan* (Atractylodes Pills).

Dosage: 6-10g

Method of use: Decoct in water and administer internally.

Cautions & contraindications: This medicinal is contraindicated in case of yin vacuity internal heat or qi vacuity with profuse perspiration.

Herba Agastachis Seu Pogostemi (*Huo Xiang*)

Nature & flavor: Acrid and slightly warm

Channel entry: Spleen, stomach, and lung channels

Functions: Aromatically penetrates and transforms dampness, effuses the exterior and resolves summerheat, opens the stomach and stops vomiting

Indications:

1. Used for dampness obstructing the middle burner with symptoms of stomach duct and abdominal distention and fullness, devitalized eating and drinking, nausea and vomiting, Herba Agastachis Seu Pogostemi is commonly combined with Rhizoma Atractylodis (*Cang Zhu*) and Cortex Magnoliae Officinalis (*Hou Po*) as in *Bu Huan Jin Zheng Qi San* (More Precious than Gold Correcting the Qi Powder).

2. Used for summerheat month external contraction wind cold or internal damage by uncooked and chilled foods and drinks resulting in cold and heat, headache, chest oppression, abdominal distention, nausea, vomiting, and diarrhea, Herba Agastachis Seu Pogostemi is commonly combined with Folium Perillae Frutescentis (*Zi Su*), Rhizoma Pinelliae Ternatae (*Ban Xia*) and Cortex Magnoliae Officinalis (*Hou Po*) as in *Huo Xiang Zheng Qi San* (Agastaches Correct the Qi Powder). For summer and fall damage due to summerheat with dizziness, chest oppression, nausea, and stickiness and sliminess within the mouth, Herba Agastachis Seu Pogostemi can be combined with Herba Eupatorii Fortunei (*Pei Lan*) and Herba Menthae Haplocalycis (*Bo He*) infused in water and administered. For this, fresh Herba Agastachis Seu Pogostemi's effect is better.

3. Used for vomiting and spitting conditions. This medicinal is most suitable for vomiting and spitting due to spleen-stomach dampness and turbidity, for which it is commonly combined with Rhizoma Pinelliae Ternatae (*Ban Xia*). For other kinds of vomiting and spitting, it can also be used depending on the condition. For instance, for damp heat, it may be used in combination with Rhizoma Coptidis Chinensis (*Huang Lian*) and Caulis Bambusae In Taeniis (*Zhu Ru*). For spleen-stomach vacuity weakness, it may be combined with Radix Codonopsitis Pilosulae (*Dang Shen*) and Radix Glycyrrhizae (*Gan Cao*). For nausea and vomiting during pregnancy, it is commonly combined with Fructus Amomi (*Sha Ren*).

Dosage: 6-10g. Use double this amount when using the fresh herb.

Method of use: Decoct in water and administer internally. It is not appropriate to decoct this ingredient for a long time.

Fructus Amomi (*Sha Ren*)

Nature & flavor: Acrid and warm

Channel entry: Spleen and stomach

Functions: Transforms dampness and opens the stomach, warms the spleen and stops diarrhea, rectifies the qi and quiets the fetus

Indications:

1. Used for dampness obstructing the middle burner and qi stagnation with stomach duct and abdominal distention and fullness, devitalized eating and drinking, vomiting and spitting, and diarrhea. If categorized as damp obstruction, Fructus Amomi is commonly combined with Cortex Magnoliae Officinalis (*Hou Po*) and Rhizoma Atractylodis (*Cang Zhu*). If there is qi stagnation and food accumulation, it can be combined with Radix Auklandiae Lappae (*Mu Xiang*) and Fructus Immaturus Citri Aurantii (*Zhi Shi*) as in *Xiang Sha Zhi Zhu Wan* (Auklandia & Amomum Aurantium & Atractylodes Pills). If there is spleen vacuity with qi stagnation, Fructus Amomi is commonly combined with Radix Codonopsitis Pilosulae (*Dang Shen*) and Rhizoma Atractylodis Macrocephalae (*Bai Zhu*) as in *Xiang Sha Liu Jun Zi Tang* (Auklandia & Amomum Six Gentlemen Decoction).

2. Used for spleen vacuity cold and dampness accumulation and stagnation diarrhea, Fructus Amomi can be powdered and taken alone washed down with water or may be used with dry Rhizoma Zingiberis (*Gan Jiang*), Radix Lateralis Praeparatus Aconiti Carmichaeli (*Fu Zi*), and Semen Myristicae Fragrantis (*Rou Dou Kou*).

3. Used for nausea during pregnancy and fetal stirring restlessness, Fructus Amomi is commonly combined with Rhizoma Atractylodis Macrocephalae (*Bai Zhu*), Caulis Perillae Frutescentis (*Su Gen*), and Ramulus Loranthi Seu Visci (*Sang Ji Sheng*).

Dosage: 3-6g

Method of use: Decoct in water and administer internally. It should be added later.

Herba Eupatorii Fortunei (*Pei Lan*)

Nature & flavor: Acrid and level

Channel entry: Spleen and stomach

Functions: Aromatically penetrates and transforms dampness, arouses the spleen and opens the stomach, effuses the exterior and resolves summerheat

Indications:

1. Used for damp accumulation obstructing the center with stomach duct glomus, nausea and vomiting, a sweet taste and slimy feeling in the mouth, bad breath, profuse saliva, Herba Eupatorii Fortunei can be combined with Rhizoma Coptidis Chinensis (*Huang Lian*).

2. Used for summerheat dampness external conditions with head distention and chest oppression, Herba Eupatorii can be combined with Talcum (*Hua Shi*).

Dosage: 6-12g. When used fresh, 15-30g.

Method of use: Decoct in water and administer internally. It is not appropriate to decoct this ingredient for a long time.

Fructus Cardamomi (*Bai Dou Kou*)

Nature & flavor: Acrid and warm

Channel entry: Lung, spleen, and stomach

Functions: Transforms dampness and disperses glomus, moves the qi and warms the center, opens the stomach and disperses food

Indications: Used for various types of chest and abdominal fullness and oppression, vomiting, and diarrhea. For the treatment of qi stagnation and damp obstruction with chest and abdominal fullness and oppression, vomiting, and diarrhea, Fructus Cardamomi can be combined with Fructus Amomi (*Sha Ren*). For the treatment of spleen and stomach vacuity weakness loss of movement resulting in turbid dampness collecting and obstructing and symptoms of chest and abdominal fullness and discomfort, burping, nausea, vomiting, and diarrhea, Fructus Cardamomi can be combined with Pericarpium Citri Reticulatae (*Chen Pi*). For the treatment of stomach duct and abdominal fullness and scanty eating from cold dampness or food stagnation, Fructus Cardamomi can be combined with Herba Agastachis Seu Pogostemi (*Huo Xiang*).

Dosage: 3-6g

Method of administration: Decoct in water and administer internally, adding later.

C. Water-disinhibiting, dampness-percolating medicinals

Sclerotium Poriae Cocos (*Fu Ling*)

Nature & flavor: Sweet, bland, and level

Channel entry: Heart, spleen, and kidneys

Functions: Disinhibits water and percolates dampness, fortifies the spleen and supplements the center, stabilizes the heart and quiets the spirit

Indications:

1. Used for inhibited urination, water swelling, phlegm rheum and other water dampness collecting and stagnating conditions, Sclerotium Poriae Cocos is commonly combined with Sclerotium Polypori Umbellati (*Zhu Ling*) and Rhizoma Alismatis (*Ze Xie*) as in *Wu Ling San* (Five [Ingredients] Poria Powder). Because Sclerotium Poriae Cocos's nature is level and harmonious, it can be used for either damp heat or cold dampness conditions when combined with other appropriate medicinals following the condition. If there is damp heat, Sclerotium Poriae Cocos is commonly combined with Semen Plantaginis (*Che Qian Zi*) and Caulis Akebiae (*Mu Tong*). If there is cold dampness, it is often combined with Radix Lateralis Praeparatus Aconiti Carmichaeli (*Fu Zi*) and dry Rhizoma Zingiberis (*Gan Jiang*). For phlegm rheum collecting internally resulting in dizziness, heart palpitations, and cough, Sclerotium Poriae Cocos is commonly combined with Ramulus Cinnamomi Cassiae (*Gui Zhi*) and Rhizoma Atractylodis Macrocephalae (*Bai Zhu*) as in *Ling Gui Zhu Gan Tang* (Poria, Cinnamon, Atractylodes & Licorice Decoction).

2. Used for spleen vacuity bodily fatigue, decreased eating, and loose stools, Sclerotium Poriae Cocos is commonly combined with Radix Codonopsitis Pilosulae (*Dang Shen*), Rhizoma Atractylodis Macrocephalae (*Bai Zhu*), and Radix Glycyrrhizae (*Gan Cao*) as in *Si Jun Zi Tang* (Four Gentlemen Decoction).

3. Used for heart-spleen insufficiency fright palpitations and insomnia, Sclerotium Poriae Cocos is commonly combined with Radix Codonopsitis Pilosulae (*Dang Shen*), Arillus Euphoriae Longanae (*Long Yan Rou*), and Semen Zizyphi Spinosae (*Suan Zao Ren*) as in

Gui Pi Tang (Return the Spleen Decoction). When used for phlegm turbidity obstructing internally or heart-kidney not interacting fright palpitations and insomnia, Sclerotium Poriae Cocos is commonly combined with Rhizoma Acori Graminei (*Shi Chang Pu*) and Radix Polygalae Tenuifoliae (*Yuan Zhi*) as in *An Shen Ding Zhi Wan* (Quiet the Spirit & Stabilize the Will Pills).

Dosage: 10-30g

Method of use: Decoct in water and administer internally.

Note: Cortex Sclerotii Poriae Cocos (*Fu Ling Pi*) has the same nature and flavor as Sclerotium Poriae Cocos. However, it is more effective for disinhibiting water and dispersing swelling, conducting and moving water dampness in the skin. Therefore, it can be used for the treatment of skin water swellling. Its dose is the same as Sclerotium Poriae Cocos.

Sclerotium Polypori Umbellati (*Zhu Ling*)

Nature & flavor: Sweet, bland, and level

Channel entry: Kidneys and urinary bladder

Functions: Disinhibits water and percolates dampness

Indications: Used for inhibited urination, water swelling, diarrhea, strangury and turbid urine, and abnormal vaginal discharge, Sclerotium Polypori Umbellati is commonly combined with Sclerotium Poriae Cocos (*Fu Ling*) and Rhizoma Alismatis (*Ze Xie*) as in *Si Ling San* (Four [Ingredients] Poria Powder) and *Zhu Ling Tang* (Polyporus Decoction). This ingredient's sweet, bland, seeping, and charging action of disinhibiting water is stronger than that of Sclerotium Poriae Cocos. However, it has no power to supplement and boost the heart and spleen. It can be used in combination with other medicinals to treat any kind of water dampness stagnation and retention.

Dosage: 10-15g

Method of use: Decoct in water and administer internally.

Rhizoma Alismatis (*Ze Xie*)

Nature & flavor: Sweet, bland, and cold

Channel entry: Kidneys and urinary bladder

Functions: Disinhibits water, percolates dampness, and discharges heat

Indications: Used for inhibited urination, water swelling, diarrhea, strangury and turbid urination, abnormal vaginal discharge, and phlegm rheum conditions. Rhizoma Alismatis's sweet, bland, dampness-percolating and water-disinhibiting action is the same as that of Sclerotium Poriae Cocos (*Fu Ling*) and can be used for various types of water dampness conditions. Because its nature tends towards being cold, it is able to discharge heat from the kidneys and urinary bladder. Therefore, it is especially appropriate for lower burner damp heat. For the treatment of inhibited urination and water swelling, Rhizoma Alismatis is commonly combined with Sclerotium Poriae Cocos and Sclerotium Polypori Umbellati (*Zhu Ling*) as in *Zhu Ling Tang* (Polyporus Decoction). For the treatment of phlegm rheum resulting in dizziness, Rhizoma Alismatis is often used in combination with Rhizoma Atractylodis Macrocephalae (*Bai Zhu*) as in *Ze Xie Tang* (Alisma Decoction).

Dosage: 5-15g

Method of use: Decoct in water and administer internally. This medicinal is typically used stir-fried in salt water.

Cautions & contraindications: Use of excessively large doses of this medicinal can result in slippery essence, *i.e.*, involuntary seminal emission.

Semen Plantaginis (*Che Qian Zi*)

Nature & flavor: Sweet and slightly cold

Channel entry: Kidneys, liver, and lungs

Functions: Disinhibits water and frees the flow of strangury, percolates dampness and stops diarrhea, clears the liver and brightens the eyes, clears the lungs and transforms phlegm

Indications:

1. Used for water swelling and inhibited urination or urinary strangury, dribbling, astringency, and pain, Semen Plantaginis is commonly combined with Caulis Akebiae (*Mu Tong*) and Talcum (*Hua Shi*) as in *Ba Zheng San* (Eight [Ingredients] Correcting Powder).

2. Used for summerheat dampness diarrhea. Semen Plantaginis is able to disinhibit urination and replete the stools in the treatment of summer and fall damp exuberance leading to watery diarrhea. In that case, Semen Plantaginis is commonly combined with Herba Agastachis Seu Pogostemi (*Huo Xiang*) and Sclerotium Poriae Cocos (*Fu Ling*) as in *Che Qian Zi San* (Plantago Powder).

3. Used for red eyes, internal obstruction of vision, and dimmed vision. For the treatment of liver heat red, swollen, painful eyes, Semen Plantaginis is often combined with Flos Chrysanthemi Morifolii (*Ju Hua*) and Radix Gentianae Scabrae (*Long Dan Cao*). For the treatment of enduring internal obstruction of vision due to liver-kidney yin vacuity, Semen Plantaginis is commonly combined with uncooked Radix Rehmanniae (*Sheng Di*), Tuber Ophiopogonis Japonici (*Mai Men Dong*), and Fructus Lycii Chinensis (*Gou Qi Zi*).

4. Used for lung heat cough with profuse phlegm, Semen Plantaginis can be combined with Radix Platycodi Grandiflori (*Jie Geng*) and Semen Pruni Armeniacae (*Xing Ren*).

Dosage: 10-15g

Method administration: Decoct in water and administer internally. Wrap during decoction. For disinhibiting urination and stopping diarrhea, use stir-fried. For transforming phlegm, use uncooked.

Caulis Akebiae (*Mu Tong*)

Nature & flavor: Bitter and cold

Channel entry: Heart, small intestine, and urinary bladder

Functions: Disinhibits water and frees the flow of strangury, discharges heat, frees the flow of the breast milk

Indications:

1. Used for urinary bladder damp heat with short, reddish urination, strangury, dribbling, astringency, and pain or for heart fire flaring upward with heart vexation, reddish urination, etc. Caulis Akebiae is commonly combined with Semen Plantaginis (*Che Qian*

Zi), uncooked Radix Rehmanniae (*Sheng Di*), and Folium Bambusae (*Zhu Ye*) as in *Ba Zheng San* (Eight [Ingredients] Correcting Powder) and *Dao Chi San* (Abduct the Red Powder).

2. Used for postpartum scanty lactation, Caulis Akebiae is commonly combined with Medulla Tetrapancis Papyriferi (*Tong Cao*), Radix Echinposis Seu Rhapontici (*Lou Lu*), Semen Vaccariae Segetalis (*Wang Bu Liu Xing*), and pig's feet.

Dosage: 3-10g

Method of use: Decoct in water and administer internally.

Cautions & contraindications: It has been reported in the journal literature that large doses of this medicinal (*i.e.*, 60g) can result in acute kidney failure. Therefore, one should not use too large a dose of this ingredient. It should be used cautiously in pregnant women.

Herba Lysimachiae (*Jin Qian Cao*)

Nature & flavor: Sweet, bland, and level

Channel entry: Liver, gallbladder, kidneys, and urinary bladder

Functions: Disinhibits water, frees the flow of strangury, and expels stones, eliminates dampness and recedes jaundice, resolves toxins and disperses swelling

Indications:

1. Used for heat strangury, stone strangury, and sand strangury. This ingredient is an essential one in the treatment of calculi of the liver, gallbladder, kidneys, bladder, and urinary tract. It can be drunk alone as a beverage tea after decoction of large doses or it can be combined with Spora Lygodii (*Hai Jin Sha*) and Endothelium Corneum Gigeriae Galli (*Ji Nei Jin*).

2. Used for damp heat jaundice, Herba Lysimachiae is commonly combined with Herba Artemisiae Capillaris (*Yin Chen Hao*) and Fructus Gardeniae Jasminoidis (*Zhi Zi*).

3. Used for clove sores, swelling, and toxins, Herba Lysimachiae can be used fresh. In this case, the herb is pounded and the juice obtained and taken. For the treatment of injury due to scalds and burns, the juice of the fresh herb can be applied externally.

Dosage: 30-60g. If used alone, 120-150g. Increase this dose to 150-300g if used fresh. Externally, use a suitable amount.

Method of use: Decoct in water and administer internally.

Herba Artemisiae Capillaris (*Yin Chen Hao*)

Nature & flavor: Bitter and slightly cold

Channel entry: Spleen, stomach, liver, and gallbladder

Functions: Clears and disinhibits dampness and heat, disinhibits the gallbladder and recedes jaundice

Indications: Used for damp heat jaundice with symptoms of yellowing of the body and eyes which are bright and fresh in color, fever, and short, reddish urination, Herba Artemisiae Capillaris is commonly combined with Fructus Gardeniae Jasminoidis (*Zhi Zi*) and Radix Et Rhizoma Rhei (*Da Huang*). This is then called *Yin Chen Hao Tang* (Capillaris Decoction). For those categorized as cold damp jaundice with a dull, dark yellow color, reduced intake of food, epigastric oppression, lassitude of the spirit, and fear of cold, Herba Artemisiae Capillaris can be combined with Radix Lateralis Praeparatus Aconiti Carmichaeli (*Fu Zi*) and dry Rhizoma Zingiberis (*Gan Jiang*) as in *Yin Chen Si Ni Tang* (Capillaris Four Counterflows Decoction).

Dosage: 15-30g

Method of use: Decoct in water and administer internally.

Talcum (*Hua Shi*)

Nature & flavor: Sweet, bland, and cold

Channel entry: Stomach and urinary bladder

Functions: Disinhibits urination and frees the flow of strangury, clears heat and resolves summerheat, dispels dampness and constrains sores

Indications:

1. Used for lower burner damp heat with heat strangury, stone strangury, or hot, astringent,

painful urination, Talcum is commonly combined with Semen Abutiloni Seu Malvae (*Dong Kui Zi*).

2. Used for summerheat dampness fever, vexatious thirst, and difficult urination, Talcum is commonly combined with Radix Glycyrrhizae (*Gan Cao*) as in *Liu Yi San* (Six [to] One Powder).

3. Used for eczema, damp sores, and prickly heat, Talcum can be used alone as a powder applied externally or combined with powdered Cortex Phellodendri (*Huang Bai*) and Alum (*Ming Fan*) and applied externally.

Dosage: 10-15g. For urinary retention, one can use up to 24-30g. Externally, use a suitable amount.

Method of use: Decoct in water and administer internally. Place in a cotton bag during decoction. Powder for external application.

Semen Coicis Lachryma-jobi (*Yi Yi Ren*)

Nature & flavor: Sweet, bland, and cool

Channel entry: Spleen, lungs, and kidneys

Functions: Fortifies the spleen and percolates dampness, eliminates impediment and stops thirst, clears heat and expels pus

Indications:

1. Used for spleen vacuity damp encumberance diarrhea, Semen Coicis Lachryma-jobi is commonly combined with Rhizoma Atractylodis Macrocephalae (*Bai Zhu*) and Sclerotium Poriae Cocos (*Fu Ling*).

2. Used for external contraction of wind dampness with mild, generalized body pain, slight aversion to wind, and fever that worsens in the afternoon, Semen Coicis Lachryma-jobi can be combined with Herba Ephedrae (*Ma Huang*), Semen Pruni Armeniacae (*Xing Ren*), and Radix Glycyrrhizae (*Gan Cao*). This is then called *Ma Xing Yi Gan Tang* (Ephedra, Armeniaca, Coix & Licorice Decoction).

3. Used for damp heat impediment pain of the lower extremities, Semen Coicis Lachryma-jobi is commonly combined with Cortex Phellodendri (*Huang Bai*), Radix Achyranthis Bidentatae (*Niu Xi*), and Fructus Chaenomelis Lagenariae (*Mu Gua*). This is then called *Si Miao San* (Four Wonders Powder).

4. Used for lung abscesses, Semen Coicis Lachryma-jobi can be combined with Rhizoma Phragmitis Communis (*Lu Gen*), Semen Benincasae Hispidae (*Dong Gua Ren*), and Semen Pruni Persicae (*Tao Ren*).

5. Used for intestinal abscesses, Semen Coicis Lachryma-jobi can be combined with Herba Patriniae Heterophyllae Cum Radice (*Bai Jiang Cao*) and Cortex Radicis Moutan (*Dan Pi*).

Dosage: 10-30g

Method of use: Decoct in water and administer internally. For disinhibiting damp heat, use uncooked. Use stir-fried for supplementing the spleen and stopping diarrhea.

Semen Benincasae Hispidae (*Dong Gua Ren*)

Nature & flavor: Sweet and slightly cold

Channel entry: Lungs, stomach, large intestine, and small intestine

Functions: Moistens the lungs, transforms phlegm, disperses welling abscesses, and disinhibits water

Indications:

1. Used for thirsting and wasting with polyuria, Semen Benincasae Hispidae can be combined with Tuber Asparagi Cochinensis (*Tian Men Dong*), and Rhizoma Coptidis Chinensis (*Huang Lian*).

2. Used for lung abscess, Semen Benincasae Hispidae can be combined with Radix platycodi Grandiflori (*Jie Geng*), Herba Houttuyniae Cordatae Cum Radice (*Yu Xing Cao*), and Flos Lonicerae Japonicae (*Jin Yin Hua*).

3. Used for intestinal abscess, Semen Benincasae Hispidae can be combined with Radix Et Rhizoma Rhei (*Da Huang*) and Cortex Radicis Moutan (*Dan Pi*).

4. For lower burner damp heat abnormal vaginal discharge, Semen Benincasae Hispidae can be combined with Cortex Phellodendri (*Huang Bai*) and Rhizoma Dioscoreae Hypoglaucae (*Bei Xie*).

Dosage: 15-30g

Method of use: Decoct in water and administer internally.

Medulla Tetrapanacis Papyriferi (*Tong Cao*)

Nature & flavor: Sweet, bland, and slightly cold

Channel entry: Lungs and stomach

Functions: Clears heat and disinhibits urination, frees the flow of qi and descends the breast milk

Indications:

1. Used for damp heat reddish urine, strangury disease, astringency and pain, Medulla Tetrapanacis Papyriferi can be combined with Herba Dianthi (*Qu Mai*).

2. Used for water swelling and scanty urination, this medicinal can be combined with Pericarpium Arecae Catechu (*Da Fu Pi*).

3. Used for non-descension of breast milk, Medulla Tetrapanacis Papyriferi is commonly combined with Squama Manitis Pentadactylis (*Chuan Shan Jia*). If due to qi and blood insufficiency, one can add Radix Angelicae Sinensis (*Dang Gui*), Radix Astragali Membranacei (*Huang Qi*), and Radix Ligustici Wallichii (*Chuan Xiong*).

Dosage: 6-10g

Method of use: Decoct in water and administer internally.

Cautions & contraindications: Use cautiously in case of qi and yin vacuities. Use cautiously in pregnant women.

Medulla Junci Effusi (*Deng Xin Cao*)

Nature & flavor: Sweet, bland, and slightly cold

Channel entry: Heart, lungs, and small intestine

Functions: Clears heart fire, disinhibits urination

Indications: Used for heart vexation, insomnia, scanty, painful astringent urination, and sores in the mouth and on the tongue due to heart fire being transferred to the small intestine, Medulla Junci Effusi can be combined with Herba Lophatheri Gracilis (*Dan Zhu Ye*) and Talcum (*Hua Shi*).

Dosage: 3-6g

Method of use: Decoct in water and administer internally.

Herba Dianthi (*Qu Mai*)

Nature & flavor: Bitter and cold

Channel entry: Heart, kidneys, small intestine, and urinary bladder

Functions: Disinhibits urination and frees the flow of strangury, breaks the blood and frees the flow of menstruation

Indications:

1. Used for hot strangury with burning heat, scanty urination, astringency, and pain, Herba Dianthi can be combined with Talcum (*Hua Shi*) and Fructus Gardeniae Jasminoidis (*Zhi Zi*). If accompanied by blood heat hematuria, add Rhizoma Imperatae Cylindricae (*Bai Mao Gen*) and Herba Cephalanoploris (*Xiao Ji*). For damp heat brewing and congealing stones in the urinary tract, Herba Dianthi can be combined with Spora Lygodii Japonici (*Hai Jin Sha*).

2. Used for blocked menstruation due to blood stasis, Herba Dianthi can be combined with Radix Salviae Miltiorrhizae (*Dan Shen*).

Dosage: 10-30g

Method of use: Decoct in water and administer internally.

Cautions & contraindications: Use cautiously in pregnant women.

Fructus Kochiae Scopariae (*Di Fu Zi*)

Nature & flavor: Acrid, bitter, and cold

Channel entry: Urinary bladder

Functions: Clears heat and disinhibits dampness, dispels wind and stops itching

Indications:

1. Used for damp heat in the lower burner resulting in urinary astringency and pain, genital itching, and abnormal vaginal discharge. For urinary astringency and pain, Fructus Kochiae Scopariae can be combined with Sclerotium Poriae Cocos (*Fu Ling*), Medulla Tetrapanacis Papyriferi (*Tong Cao*), and Herba Dianthi (*Qu Mai*). For genital itching and

abnormal vaginal discharge, Fructus Kochiae Scopariae is commonly combined with Radix Sophorae Flavescentis (*Ku Shen*) and Semen Cnidii Monnieri (*She Chuang Zi*).

2. Used for wind rash, eczema, and itching of the skin due to either damp heat or wind heat, Fructus Kochiae Scopariae can be combined with uncooked Radix Rehmanniae (*Sheng Di*) and Cortex Radicis Dictamni Dasycarpi (*Bai Xian Pi*).

Dosage: 10-15g. Externally, use a suitable amount.

Method of use: Decoct in water and administer internally or use as a fumigation and wash to the affected area.

Herba Polygoni Avicularis (*Bian Xu*)

Nature & flavor: Bitter and slightly cold

Channel entry: Urinary bladder

Functions: Disinhibits urination and frees the flow of strangury, kills worms, stops itching

Indications:

1. Used for urinary bladder heat strangury with short, reddish urination, dribbling and dripping, astringency, and pain, Herba Polygoni Avicularis is commonly combined with Herba Dianthi (*Qu Mai*) and Semen Plantaginis (*Che Qian Zi*).

2. Used for pinworms, Herba Polygoni Avicularis can be combined with Semen Torreyae Grandis (*Fei Zi*), Radix Stemonae (*Bai Bu*), and Semen Arecae Catechu (*Bing Lang*).

3. Used for lower burner damp heat genital itching, Herba Polygoni Avicularis can be combined with Fructus Kochiae Scopariae (*Di Fu Zi*) to use as an external wash.

Dosage: 10-15g. Externally, use a suitable amount.

Method of use: Decoct in water and administer or use as a fumigation and wash applied externally to the affected area.

Semen Abutiloni Seu Malvae (*Dong Kui Zi*)

Nature & flavor: Sweet, astringent, and cool

Channel entry: Large intestine, small intestine, and urinary bladder

Functions: Clears heat and disinhibits urination, disperses swelling

Indications:

1. Used for urinary tract infection, urinary block, water swelling, and oral thirst. For the treatment of postpartum urinary retention and water swelling, Semen Abutiloni Seu Malvae can be combined with Sclerotium Poriae Cocos (*Fu Ling*). For the treatment of urinary tract stones, Semen Abutiloni Seu Malvae can be combined with Semen Plantaginis (*Che Qian Zi*) and Spora Lygodii (*Hai Jin Sha*). For the treatment of urinary astringency, frequency, and pain in children, this medicinal can be combined with Caulis Akebiae (*Mu Tong*).

2. Used for scanty lactation and breast distention and pain due to stagnant qi, Semen Abutiloni Seu Malvae can be combined with Fructus Amomi (*Sha Ren*).

Dosage: 10-15g

Method of use: Decoct in water and administer internally

Cautions & contraindications: This medicinal is contraindicated in case of spleen vacuity loose stools and diarrhea. Use cautiously in pregnant women.

Rhizoma Dioscoreae Hypoglaucae (*Bei Xie*)

Nature & flavor: Bitter and level

Channel entry: Liver, stomach, and urinary bladder

Functions: Disinhibits dampness and dispels turbidity, dispels wind and frees the flow of impediment

Indications:

1. Used for turbid dampness and heat in the lower burner resulting in turbid strangury and abnormal vaginal discharge, Rhizoma Dioscoreae Hypoglaucae is commonly combined with Cortex Phellodendri (*Huang Bai*), Rhizoma Acori Graminei (*Shi Chang Pu*), and

Semen Plantaginis (*Che Qian Zi*) as in *Bei Xie Fen Qing Yin* (Dioscorea Hypoglauca Divide the Clear Drink).

2. Used for wind damp and damp heat impediment pain, low back and knee aching and pain, and numbness of the lower extremities, Rhizoma Dioscoreae Hypoglaucae is commonly combined with Radix Clematidis Chinesis (*Wei Ling Xian*) and Radix Achyranthis Bidentatae (*Niu Xi*).

3. Used for damp heat sores and toxins, Rhizoma Dioscoreae Hypoglaucae is commonly combined with Semen Coicis Lachryma-jobi (*Yi Yi Ren*) and Cortex Phellodendri (*Huang Bai*).

Dosage: 10-15g

Method of use: Decoct in water and administer internally.

Semen Phaseoli Calcarati (*Chi Xiao Dou*)

Nature & flavor: Sweet, sour, and level

Channel entry: Heart and small intestine

Functions: Disinhibits water and disperses swelling, resolves toxins and expels pus

Indications:

1. Used for water swelling, distention, and fullness and leg qi superficial edema, Semen Phaseoli Calcarati are commonly combined with carp, cooked, and eaten. For vacuity edema, it is cooked into soup with peanuts and Fructus Zizyphi Jujubae (*Da Zao*) and eaten for an extended period of time.

2. Used for damp heat resulting in jaundice with reddish urine, Semen Phaseoli Calcarati can be combined with Herba Ephedrae (*Ma Huang*), Fructus Forsythiae Suspensae (*Lian Qiao*), and Cortex Radicis Mori Albi (*Sang Bai Pi*).

In addition, Semen Phaseoli Calcarati can also be used as an external application for the treatment of welling abscess swelling, sores, and toxins.

Dosage: 15-30g. Externally, use a suitable amount.

Method of administration: Decoct in water and administer internally. For external application, grind into powder, mix with water, and apply to the affected area..

6

Interior-warming medicinals

Medicinals which are able to warm and scatter interior cold and thus treat interior cold conditions are called interior-warming medicinals. Due to their nature being acrid and hot, this class of medicinals is able to dispel and scatter yin cold located in the interior and restore the body's yang qi. They are mainly suitable for the use in cold evils internally assailing with spleen yang smothered and encumbered resulting in stomach duct and abdominal chilly pain, vomiting and spitting, and diarrhea as well as for yang qi decline and weakness with yin cold internally exuberant resulting in fear of cold, chilled limbs, a somber white facial complexion, clear, long urination, a pale tongue, and a fine pulse. Some of these medicinals have the power to return yang and stem counterflow and are thus suitable for using in perishing yang.

Depending on different conditions, interior-warming medicinals should be combined with different medicinals. If there is external cold internally assailing with a simultaneous exterior pattern, they should be combined with exterior-resolving medicinals. If there is cold coagulation and qi stagnation, they should be combined with qi-moving medicinals. And if yang vacuity is engendering cold, they should be combined with warming and supplementing medicinals.

Because this group of medicinals is acrid, warm, and drying, they easily invigorate fire and damage yin. Therefore, these medicinals should be used cautiously or are contraindicated in those categorized as heat patterns, yin vacuity patterns, or in pregnant women.

Radix Lateralis Praeparatus Aconiti Carmichaeli (*Fu Zi*)

Nature & flavor: Acrid and greatly hot. Has toxins.

Channel entry: Heart, kidneys, and spleen

Functions: Returns yang and stems counterflow, supplements fire and invigorates yang, scatters cold and stops pain

Indications:

1. Used for perishing yang conditions with symptoms of chilly sweating, spontaneous perspiration, reversal counterflow of the four extremities, and a faint pulse on the verge

of expiry, Radix Lateralis Praeparatus Aconiti Carmichaeli is commonly combined with dry Rhizoma Zingiberis (*Gan Jiang*) as in *Si Ni Tang* (Four Counterflows Decoction).

2. Used for yang vacuity patterns. For kidney yang insufficiency fear of cold, chilled limbs, impotence, and frequent urination, Radix Lateralis Praeparatus Aconiti Carmichaeli is commonly combined with Cortex Cinnamomi Cassiae (*Rou Gui*), cooked Radix Rehmanniae (*Shu Di*), and Fructus Corni Officinalis (*Shan Zhu Yu*) as in *Shen Qi Wan* (Kidney Qi Pills). For devitalized spleen yang stomach duct and abdominal chilly pain, torpid intake, and loose stools, this medicinal can be combined with Radix Panacis Ginseng (*Ren Shen*), Rhizoma Atractylodis Macrocephalae (*Bai Zhu*) and dry Rhizoma Zingiberis (*Gan Jiang*) as in *Fu Zi Li Zhong Wan* (Aconite Rectify the Center Pills). For heart yang decline and weakness heart palpitations, shortness of qi, *i.e.*, breath, and chest impediment chest pain, it can be combined with Radix Panacis Ginseng (*Ren Shen*) and Ramulus Cinnamomi Cassiae (*Gui Zhi*). For spleen-kidney yang vacuity inhibited urination and superficial edema of the body and limbs, it is commonly combined with Rhizoma Atractylodis Macrocephalae (*Bai Zhu*) and Sclerotium Poriae Cocos (*Fu Ling*) as in *Zhen Wu Tang* (True Warrior Decoction).

3. Used for impediment condition bone joint aching and pain all over the body categorized as cold damp tending to exuberance, Radix Lateralis Praeparatus Aconiti Carmichaeli can be combined with Ramulus Cinnamomi Cassiae (*Gui Zhi*), Rhizoma Atractylodis Macrocephalae (*Bai Zhu*), and Radix Glycyrrhizae (*Gan Cao*) as in *Gan Cao Fu Zi Tang* (Licorice & Aconite Decoction).

In addition, when this medicinal is combined with Radix Astragali Membranacei (*Huang Qi*), as in *Qi Fu Tang* (Astragalus & Aconite Decoction), it is able to treat yang vacuity spontaneous perspiration. When it is combined with Herba Ephedrae (*Ma Huang*) and Herba Asari Cum Radice (*Xi Xin*), as in *Ma Huang Fu Zi Xi Xin Tang* (Ephedra, Aconite & Asarum Decoction), it can be used for yang vacuity external contraction wind cold.

Dosage: 3-12g.

Method of use: Decoct in water and administer internally. When used in decoctions, it should be decocted first for 30-60 minutes.

Cautions & contraindications: This ingredient has toxins. When taken internally in too large an amount or if boiled for too short a time, it may easily lead to poisoning. It is contraindicated in pregnant women, those with yang exuberance, or those with yin vacuity.

Dry Rhizoma Zingiberis (*Gan Jiang*)

Nature & flavor: Acrid and hot

Channel entry: Spleen, stomach, heart, and lungs

Functions: Warms the center and scatters cold, warms the lungs and transforms rheum

Indications:

1. Used for spleen-stomach vacuity cold with symptoms of stomach duct and abdominal chilly pain, vomiting, diarrhea, and devitalized eating and drinking, dry Rhizoma Zingiberis is commonly combined with Radix Panacis Ginseng (*Ren Shen*), Rhizoma Atractylodis Macrocephalae (*Bai Zhu*), and Radix Glycyrrhizae (*Gan Cao*) as in *Li Zhong Wan* (Rectify the Center Pills). For vomiting and diarrhea due to cold evils striking straight away the stomach bowel, dry Rhizoma Zingiberis can be used alone, in which case it is powdered, mixed with warm water, and taken internally. Or it may be combined with Rhizoma Pinelliae Ternatae (*Ban Xia*) as in *Ban Xia Gan Jiang San* (Pinellia & Dry Ginger Powder).

2. Used for cold rheum deep-lying in the lungs with symptoms of cough, qi panting, a cold form and chilly upper back, and profuse, clear, watery phlegm, dry Rhizoma Zingiberis is commonly combined with Herba Ephedrae (*Ma Huang*), Herba Asari Cum Radice (*Xi Xin*), and Fructus Schisandrae Chinensis (*Wu Wei Zi*) as in *Xiao Qing Long Tang* (Minor Blue-green Dragon Decoction).

In addition, combining this medicinal with Radix Lateralis Preaparatus Aconiti Carmichaeli (*Fu Zi*) is able to increase the yang-returning, counterflow-stemming power of Radix Lateralis Praeparatus Aconiti Carmichaeli at the same time as reducing Aconite's toxicity.

When this ingredient is stir-fried till its exterior becomes slightly black while its interior is still yellow in color, this is called blast-fried Rhizoma Zingiberis (*Pao Jiang*). It's effect of warming the interior is weaker than that of dry Rhizoma Zingiberis. However, it is longer, *i.e.*, more effective, for warming the channels and stopping bleeding. It is appropriate to use in vacuity cold natured bleeding, such as spitting blood, hemafecia, and flooding and leaking accompanied by lack of warmth in the hands and feet, a pale tongue, and a fine pulse. It can also be used for spleen-stomach vacuity cold abdominal pain and diarrhea and dysentery.

Dosage: 3-10g

Method of use: Decoct in water and administer internally.

Cautions & contraindications: Use cautiously in heat conditions, yin vacuity, and pregnant women.

Note: Blast-fried Rhizoma Zingiberis (*Pao Jiang*), also called *Hei Jiang*, is bitter and warm. Its scattering nature is less. Its functions are to warm the channels and stop bleeding. It mainly treats vacuity cold spitting of blood, hemafecia, and blood flooding. It is contraindicated in case of yin vacuity blood heat frenetically moving patterns of bleeding. Its dosage is 1.5-6g.

Cortex Cinnamomi Cassiae (*Rou Gui*)

Nature & flavor: Acrid, sweet, and greatly hot

Channel entry: Kidneys, spleen, heart, and liver

Functions: Supplements fire and invigorates yang, scatters cold and stops pain, warms and frees the flow of the channels and vessels

Indications:

1. Used for yang vacuity conditions. For kidney yang insufficiency fear of cold, chilled limbs, impotence, and frequent urination, Cortex Cinnamomi Cassiae is commonly combined with Radix Lateralis Preaparatus Aconiti Carmichaeli (*Fu Zi*) and cooked Radix Rehmanniae (*Shu Di*) as in *Shen Qi Wan* (Kidney Qi Pills). For spleen yang insufficiency stomach duct and abdominal chilly pain, decreased eating, and loose stools, Cortex Cinnamomi Cassiae can be combined with Radix Lateralis Praeparatus Aconiti Carmichaeli (*Fu Zi*), dry Rhizoma Zingiberis (*Gan Jiang*), and Rhizoma Atractylodis Macrocephalae (*Bai Zhu*) as in *Gui Fu Li Zhong Wan* (Cinnamon & Aconite Rectify the Center Pills).

2. Used for cold coagulation qi stagnation or cold coagulation blood stasis resulting in various types of aching and pain. For cold impediment low back pain, Cortex Cinnamomi Cassiae is commonly combined with Radix Angelicae Pubescentis (*Du Huo*), Ramulus Loranthi Seu Visci (*Sang Ji Sheng*), and Cortex Eucommiae Ulmoidis (*Du Zhong*). For women's blood cold blocked menstruation and painful menstruation, Cortex Cinnamomi Cassiae can be combined with Radix Angelicae Sinensis (*Dang Gui*), Radix Ligustici Wallichii (*Chuan Xiong*), and Flos Carthami Tinctorii (*Hong Hua*).

3. Used for sores and welling abcesses in the external medicine department categorized as qi and blood vacuity cold. For yin flat abscesses and chronic swellings with no head which are not red or hot, Cortex Cinnamomi Cassiae is commonly combined with uncooked

Radix Rehmanniae (*Shu Di*), Gelatinum Cornu Cervi (*Lu Jiao Jiao*), and Herba Ephedrae (*Ma Huang*) as in *Yang He Tang* (Yang Harmonizing Decoction). For welling abscesses and swellings which have produced pus but have not ruptured or, if after rupturing, endure without restraining and constraining, *i.e.*, closing, Cortex Cinnamomi Cassiae is commonly combined with Radix Astragali Membranacei (*Huang Qi*) and Radix Angelicae Sinensis (*Dang Gui*) as in *Tuo Li Huang Qi Tang* (Out-thrust the Interior Astragalus Decoction).

Dosage: 1-5g

Method of use: Decoct in water and administer internally. When decocted, add later. It may also be ground into powder and washed down with the rest of the decocted prescription, taking 1-2g each time.

Cautions & contraindications: Because this medicinal is acrid and hot and stirs the blood, it is contraindicated in those with yin vacuity fire effulgence, those with interior replete heat, and in pregnant women.

Fructus Evodiae Rutecarpae (*Wu Zhu Yu*)

Nature & flavor: Acrid, bitter, and hot. Has small toxins.

Channel entry: Liver, spleen, and stomach

Functions: Scatters cold, dries dampness, courses the liver, downbears counterflow, stops pain

Indications:

1. Used for interior cold patterns. For the treatment of stomach duct and abdominal chilly pain, Fructus Evodiae Rutecarpae can be combined with dry Rhizoma Zingiberis (*Gan Jiang*) and Radix Auklandiae Lappae (*Mu Xiang*). For the treatment of cold mounting abdominal pain, Fructus Evodiae Rutecarpae can be combined with Radix Linderae Strychnifoliae (*Wu Yao*), Fructus Foeniculi Vulgaris (*Xiao Hui Xiang*), and Semen Litchi Chinensis (*Li Zhi He*). For the treatment of middle burner vacuity cold or liver qi counterflowing upward resulting in headache and spitting of drool, it can be combined with Radix Panacis Ginseng (*Ren Shen*) and uncooked Rhizoma Zingiberis (*Sheng Jiang*) as in *Wu Zhu Yu Tang* (Evodia Decoction). For the treatment of spleen-kidney yang vacuity enduring diarrhea or fifth watch diarrhea, it can be combined with Fructus Psoraleae Corylifoliae (*Bu Gu Zhi*) and Semen Myrsticae Fragrantis (*Rou Dou Kou*) as in *Si Shen Wan* (Four Spirits Pills).

2. Used for cold damp leg qi aching and pain, Fructus Evodiae Rutecarpae is commonly

combined with Fructus Chaenomelis Lagenariae (*Mu Gua*) as in *Ji Ming San* (Cock Crow Powder).

3. Used for vomiting and swallowing of acid. If categorized as stomach cold, Fructus Evodiae Rutecarpae can be combined with uncooked Rhizoma Zingiberis (*Sheng Jiang*) and Rhizoma Pinelliae Ternatae (*Ban Xia*). If categorized as liver fire assailing the stomach, it can be combined with Rhizoma Coptidis Chinensis (*Huang Lian*) as in *Zuo Jin Wan* (Left Gold Pills).

In addition, when this ingredient is powdered, mixed with vinegar, and applied to the hearts, *i.e.*, centers, of the feet, it can lead fire to move downward, thus treating mouth and tongue sores. This can also be used to treat high blood pressure disease.

Dosage: 1-5g

Method of use: Decoct in water and administer internally. Externally, use a suitable amount.

Cautions & contraindications: This medicinal is contraindicated in those with yin vacuity who have heat.

Fructus Zanthoxyli Bungeani (*Chuan Jiao*)

Nature & flavor: Acrid and warm

Channel entry: Spleen, lungs, and kidneys

Functions: Warms the center and stops pain, kills worms and stops itching

Indications:

1. Used for stomach duct and abdominal chilly pain, vomiting and spitting, and diarrhea. For the treatment of spleen-stomach vacuity cold with stomach duct and abdominal pain, nausea, and vomiting, Fructus Zanthoxyli Bungeani is commonly combined with dry Rhizoma Zingiberis (*Gan Jiang*) and Radix Codonopsitis Pilosulae (*Dang Shen*). For the treatment of cold damp diarrhea, Fructus Zanthoxyli Bungeani can be combined with Rhizoma Atractylodis (*Cang Zhu*), Pericarpium Citri Reticulatae (*Chen Pi*), and Radix Auklandiae Lappae (*Mu Xiang*).

2. Used for various types of parasite and especially for roundworm abdominal pain and vomiting, Fructus Zanthoxyli Bungeani is commonly combined with Fructus Pruni Mume (*Wu Mei*) and dry Rhizoma Zingiberis (*Gan Jiang*) as in *Wu Mei Wan* (Mume Pills).

In addition, this medicinal can be used as an external wash for the treatment of itching and eczema when combined with Radix Sophorae Flavescentis (*Ku Shen*) and Fructus Kochiae Scopariae (*Di Fu Zi*).

Dosage: 2-6g. Externally, use a suitable amount.

Method of administration: Decoct in water and administer internally. Externally, decoct and use as a fumigation and wash of the affected area.

Cautions & contraindications: This medicinal is contraindicated in case of yin vacuity with heat symptoms. Use cautiously in pregnant women.

Flos Caryophylli (*Ding Xiang*)

Nature & flavor: Acrid and warm

Channel entry: Stomach, spleen, and kidneys

Functions: Warms the center and downbears counterflow, supplements the kidneys and invigorates yang

Indications:

1. Used for spleen-stomach vacuity cold nausea, vomiting, scanty eating, and heart and abdominal chilly pain, Flos Caryophylli is commonly combined with Fructus Evodiae Rutecarpae (*Wu Zhu Yu*) and dry Rhizoma Zingiberis (*Gan Jiang*) as in *Ding Yu Li Zhong Tang* (Clove & Evodia Rectify the Center Decoction) or Calyx Diospyros Khaki (*Shi Di*) and Radix Panacis Ginseng (*Ren Shen*) as in *Ding Xiang Shi Di Tang* (Clove & Persimmon Calyx Decoction).

2. Used for various kidney yang vacuity conditions. For the treatment of impotence and abnormal vaginal discharge, Flos Caryophylli can be combined with Cortex Cinnamomi Cassiae (*Rou Gui*). For the treatment of women's flooding and leaking, it may be combined with Folium Artemisiae Argyii (*Ai Ye*) and Gelatinum Corii Asini (*E Jiao*) as in *Ding Xiang Jiao Ai Tang* (Clove, Mugwort & Donkey Skin Glue Decoction).

Dosage: 1-3g

Method of use: Decoct in water and administer internally.

Cautions & contraindications: This medicinal is not appropriate for use in warm heat diseases and yin vacuity conditions.

Fructus Foeniculi Vulgaris (*Xiao Hui Xiang*)

Nature & flavor: Acrid, sweet, and warm

Channel entry: Stomach, liver, and kidneys

Functions: Scatters cold and stops pain, rectifies the qi and harmonizes the stomach

Indications:

1. Used for cold mounting abdominal pain, one-sided testicular sagging, painful menstruation, and lower abdominal chilly pain, Fructus Foeniculi Vulgaris is commonly combined with Radix Linderae Strychnifoliae (*Wu Yao*), Semen Citri Reticulatae (*Ju He*), and Semen Litchi Chinensis (*Li Zhi He*).

2. Used for stomach cold resulting in stomach duct and abdominal distention and pain, vomiting, and scanty eating, Fructus Foeniculi Vulgaris can be combined with uncooked Rhizoma Zingiberis (*Sheng Jiang*) and Cortex Magnoliae Officinalis (*Hou Po*).

Dosage: 6-10g

Method of use: Decoct in water and administer internally.

Cautions & contraindication: This medicinal is contraindicated in case of yin vacuity fire effulgence.

7

Qi-rectifying medicinals

Medicinals which regulate and rectify the qi mechanism and mainly promote the free and smooth flow of the qi's movement are called qi rectifying medicinals. Such medicinals have the effect of moving the qi and stopping pain, normalizing the flow of qi and downbearing counterflow, and breaking the qi and scattering nodulation and are suitable for use in unsmooth flow of the qi mechanism resulting in qi stagnation and qi counterflow conditions. This includes liver qi depression and stagnation flank and rib-side or breast distention and pain, mounting pain, menstrual irregularity; spleen-stomach qi stagnation stomach duct and abdominal distention and pain, burping and acid regurgitation; lung loss of diffusion and downbearing chest oppression and coughing; and stomach qi not downbearing vomiting, nausea, and hiccup.

Because the medicinals in this category are mostly acrid and dry in nature, they easily consume the qi and damage yin. Therefore, they should be used cautiously in case of qi vacuity and yin debility.

Pericarpium Citri Reticulatae (*Chen Pi*)

Nature & flavor: Acrid, bitter, and warm

Channel entry: Spleen and lungs

Functions: Rectifies the qi and harmonizes the middle, dries dampness and transforms phlegm

Indications:

1. Used for spleen-stomach qi stagnation resulting in stomach duct and abdominal distention and fullness, burping, nausea, and vomiting, Pericarpium Citri Reticulatae is commonly combined with Radix Auklandiae Lappae (*Mu Xiang*), Fructus Amomi (*Sha Ren*), and Fructus Citri Aurantii (*Zhi Ke*). If there is simultaneous spleen-stomach qi vacuity with fatigue and lack of strength, it can be combined with Radix Codonopsitis Pilosulae (*Dang Shen*), Rhizoma Atractylodis Macrocephalae (*Bai Zhu*), and Radix Glycyrrhizae (*Gan Cao*) as in *Yi Gong San* (Strange Ability Powder).

2. Used for dampness and turbidity obstructing the middle resulting in chest oppression and abdominal distention, torpid intake, fatigue, loose stools, and thick, slimy tongue fur, Pericarpium Citri Reticulatae is commonly combined with Rhizoma Atractylodis (*Cang*

Zhu) and Cortex Magnoliae Officinalis (*Hou Po*) as in *Ping Wei San* (Level the Stomach Powder).

3. Used for phlegm dampness blocking the lungs with cough and profuse phlegm, and chest and diaphragmatic fullness and oppression, Pericarpium Citri Reticulatae is commonly combined with Rhizoma Pinelliae Ternatae (*Ban Xia*) and Sclerotium Poriae Cocos (*Fu Ling*).

Dosage: 3-10g

Method of use: Decoct in water and administer internally.

Cautions & contraindications: It is not appropriate to use this medicinal if there is no qi stagnation and phlegm dampness.

Fructus Immaturus Citri Aurantii (*Zhi Shi*)

Nature & flavor: Bitter, acrid, and slightly cold

Channel entry: Spleen, stomach, and large intestine

Functions: Breaks the qi and disperses accumulations, transforms phlegm and eliminates glomus

Indications:

1. Used for accumulation and stagnation collecting internally with the qi movement suffering obstruction resulting in stomach duct and abdominal distention, fullness, aching, and pain. For food accumulation collecting and stagnating abdominal pain, constipation, putrid eructations, and bad breath, Fructus Immaturus Citri Aurantii can be combined with Fructus Crataegi (*Shan Zha*), Fructus Germinatus Hordei Vulgaris (*Mai Ya*), and Massa Medica Fermentata (*Shen Qu*). For heat binding constipation with abdominal pain, distention, and fullness, it can be combined with Cortex Magnoliae Officinalis (*Hou Po*) and Radix Et Rhizoma Rhei (*Da Huang*) as in *Xiao Cheng Qi Tang* (Minor Order the Qi Decoction). For damp heat accumulation and stagnation, diarrhea, and dysentery, and tenesmus, it can be combined with Radix Et Rhizoma Rhei (*Da Huang*), Rhizoma Coptidis Chinensis (*Huang Lian*), and Radix Scutellariae Baicalensis (*Huang Qin*) as in *Zhi Shi Dao Zhi Wan* (Immature Aurantium Abduct Stagnation Pills). For spleen vacuity loss of movement with abdominal distention after meals, Fructus Immaturus Citri Aurantii can be combined with Rhizoma Atractylodis Macrocephalae (*Bai Zhu*) as in *Zhi Zhu Wan* (Aurantium & Atractylodes Pills).

2. Used for phlegm turbidity obstructing and blocking the qi mechanism chest and

epigastric glomus and fullness. For devitalized chest yang with phlegm turbidity internally obstructing chest impediment and shortness of qi, Fructus Immaturus Citri Aurantii can be combined with Bulbus Allii (*Xie Bai*), Ramulus Cinnamomi Cassiae (*Gui Zhi*), and Fructus Trichosanthis Kirlowii (*Gua Lou*) as in *Zhi Shi Xie Bai Gui Zhi Tang* (Aurantium Immaturus, Allium & Cinnamon Twig Decoction). For dampness and phlegm obstructing the middle chest glomus and epigastric oppression, it can be combined with Pericarpium Citri Reticulatae (*Chen Pi*) and uncooked Rhizoma Zingiberis (*Sheng Jiang*) as in *Ju Zhi Jiang Tang* (Orange Peel, Aurantium Immaturus & Ginger Decoction).

In addition, Fructus Immaturus Citri Aurantii is also suitable for use in prolapse of the stomach, gastric dilation, and anal and uterine prolapse. However, in those cases, it should be combined with Radix Astragali Membranacei (*Huang Qi*) and Rhizoma Cimicifugae (*Sheng Ma*).

The fully ripe fruit of Citrus Aurantium is called Fructus Citri Aurantii (*Zhi Ke*). Its actions are the same as Fructus Immaturus Citri Aurantii but its power is more moderate. It is mainly for moving the qi, loosening the middle, and eliminating distention.

Dosage: 3-10g

Method of use: Decoct in water and administer internally.

Cautions & contraindications: This medicinal should be used cautiously in those with spleen-stomach vacuity weakness and during pregnancy.

Radix Auklandiae Lappae (*Mu Xiang*)

Nature & flavor: Acrid, bitter, and warm

Channel entry: Spleen, stomach, large intestine, and gallbladder

Functions: Moves the qi, rectifies the middle, and stops pain

Indications:

1. Used for spleen-stomach qi stagnation resulting in stomach duct and abdominal distention and pain, devitalized eating and drinking, borborygmus, and diarrhea and dysentery, Radix Auklandiae Lappae is commonly combined with Fructus Citri Aurantii (*Zhi Ke*), Fructus Meliae Toosendan (*Chuan Lian Zi*), and Rhizoma Corydalis Yanhusuo (*Yan Hu Suo*). For damp heat accumulation and stagnation in the stomach and intestines with the qi mechanism suffering obstruction and thus there is abdominal pain, diarrhea and dysentery, and tenesmus, Radix Auklandiae Lappae is commonly combined with Rhizoma Coptidis Chinensis (*Huang Lian*). This is called *Xiang Lian Wan* (Auklandia & Coptis

Pills). In the treatment of food accumulation diarrhea and dysentry, Radix Auklandiae Lappae is commonly combined with Semen Arecae Catechu (*Bing Lang*), Fructus Immaturus Citri Aurantii (*Zhi Shi*), and Radix Et Rhizoma Rhei (*Da Huang*) as in *Mu Xiang Bing Lang Wan* (Auklandia & Arecae Pills).

2. Used for spleen vacuity loss of movement with stomach duct and abdominal distention and fullness and no thought for food or drink, Radix Auklandiae Lappae can be combined with Radix Codonopsitis Pilosulae (*Dang Shen*), Rhizoma Atractylodis Macrocephalae (*Bai Zhu*), and Fructus Amomi (*Sha Ren*) as in *Xiang Sha Liu Jun Zi Tang* (Auklandia & Amomum Six Gentlemen Decoction).

In addition, this medicinal can also be used for damp heat depression and steaming and inhibition of the liver and gallbladder's coursing and discharging resulting in rib-side and flank distention and pain, a bitter taste in the mouth, and yellow tongue fur. In that case, Radix Auklandiae Lappae can be combined with Radix Bupleuri (*Chai Hu*), Tuber Curcumae (*Yu Jin*), and Fructus Citri Aurantii (*Zhi Ke*). A small amount of Radix Auklandiae Lappae may also be used along with enriching and supplementing medicinals in order to reduce their slimy, stagnating nature and thus prevent the emergence of the side effects of chest oppression, abdominal distention, and reduced desire to eat.

Dosage: 3-10g

Method of use: Decoct in water and administer internally. For moving qi stagnation, use uncooked. For stopping diarrhea, mostly use roasted. It is not appropriate to decoct this medicinal for a long time.

Cautions & contraindications: Use cautiously in cases of yin vacuity fire effulgence.

Rhizoma Cyperi Rotundi (*Xiang Fu*)

Nature & flavor: Acrid, slightly bitter, slightly sweet, and level

Channel entry: Liver and triple burner

Functions: Courses the liver and rectifies the qi, regulates the menses and stops pain

Indications:

1. Used for liver qi depression and stagnation resulting in chest, rib-side, stomach duct, and abdominal distention, fullness, aching, and pain. For the treatment of rib-side and flank aching and pain, Rhizoma Cyperi Rotundi can be combined with Radix Bupleuri (*Chai Hu*), Fructus Citri Aurantii (*Zhi Shi*), and Radix Albus Paeoniae Lactiflorae (*Bai Shao*) as in *Chai Hu Shu Gan San* (Bupleurum Course the Liver Powder). For the

treatment of liver qi assailing the stomach with stomach duct and abdominal pain, Rhizoma Cyperi Rotundi can be combined with Radix Auklandiae Lappae (*Mu Xiang*) and Fructus Citri Sacrodactylis (*Fo Shou*). For the treatment of cold mounting abdominal pain, it can be combined with Fructus Foeniculi Vulgaris (*Xiao Hui Xiang*) and Radix Linderae Strychnifoliae (*Wu Yao*). For the treatment of breast distention and pain, Rhizoma Cyperi Rotundi can be combined with Radix Bupleuri (*Chai Hu*), Fructus Trichosanthis Kirlowii (*Gua Lou*), and Folium Citri (*Ju Ye*).

2. Used for liver depression qi stagnation resulting in menstrual irregularity and menstrual movement abdominal pain, Rhizoma Cyperi Rotundi is commonly combined with Radix Angelicae Sinensis (*Dang Gui*), Radix Ligustici Wallichii (*Chuan Xiong*), and Radix Albus Paeoniae Lactiflorae (*Bai Shao*). For painful menstruation accompanied by lower abdominal chilly pain, it can be combined with Folium Artemisiae Argyii (*Ai Ye*) as in *Ai Fu Wan* (Mugwort & Cyperus Pills).

Dosage: 6-12g

Method of use: Decoct in water and administer internally. For rectifying the qi and resolving depression, use uncooked. For regulating the menses and stopping pain, one can use processed.

Cautions & contraindications: Use cautiously in cases of qi vacuity or blood heat.

Cortex Magnoliae Officinalis (*Hou Po*)

Nature & flavor: Bitter, acrid, and warm

Channel entry: Spleen, stomach, lungs, and large intestine

Functions: Moves the qi, dries dampness, disperses accumulation, levels panting

Indications:

1. Used for damp obstruction, food accumulation, and qi stagnation of various types resulting in stomach duct and abdominal distention and pain. For dampness obstructing the middle burner with abdominal distention, nausea, and vomiting, Cortex Magnoliae Officinalis can be combined with Rhizoma Atractylodis (*Cang Zhu*) and Pericarpium Citri Reticulatae (*Chen Pi*) as in *Ping Wei San* (Level the Stomach Powder). For food accumulation qi stagnation with abdominal distention and constipation, Cortex Magnoliae Officinalis can be combined with Radix Et Rhizoma Rhei (*Da Huang*) and Fructus Immaturus Citri Aurantii (*Zhi Shi*) as in *Hou Po San Wu Tang* (Magnolia Three Materials Decoction).

2. Used for damp phlegm blocking the lungs cough and qi panting, Cortex Magnoliae Officinalis can be combined with Herba Ephedrae (*Ma Huang*), Rhizoma Pinelliae Ternatae (*Ban Xia*), and Semen Pruni Armeniacae (*Xing Ren*) as in *Hou Po Ma Huang Tang* (Magnolia & Ephedra Decoction).

Dosage: 3-10g

Method of use: Decoct in water and administer internally.

Cautions & contraindications: Use cautiously in those with spleen-stomach qi vacuity.

Bulbus Allii (*Xie Bai*)

Nature & flavor: Acrid, bitter, and warm

Channel entry: Lungs, stomach, and large intestine

Functions: Frees the flow of yang and scatters nodulations, moves the qi and abducts stagnation

Indications:

1. Used for cold phlegm coagulation and stagnation and non-diffusion of chest yang resulting in chest impediment aching and pain, Bulbus Allii is commonly combined with Fructus Trichosanthis Kirlowii (*Gua Lou*) as in *Gua Lou Xie Bai Bai Jiu Tang* (Trichosanthes, Allium & White Alcohol Decoction). For qi stagnation phlegm obstruction which is relatively severe with symptoms of chest oppression, shortness of qi, and cough with profuse phlegm, Bulbus Allii can be combined with Fructus Immaturus Citri Aurantii (*Zhi Shi*) and Cortex Magnoliae Officinalis (*Hou Po*) as in *Zhi Shi Xie Bai Gui Zhi Tang* (Immature Aurantium, Allium & Cinnamon Twig Decoction). If there is simultaneous static blood obstruction and stagnation with symptoms of chest and upper back piercing pain, Bulbus Allii can be combined with Radix Salviae Miltiorrhizae (*Dan Shen*), Flos Carthami Tinctorii (*Hong Hua*), and Radix Rubrus Paeoniae Lactiflorae (*Chi Shao*).

2. Used for stomach and intestine qi stagnation diarrhea and dysentry tenesmus, Bulbus Allii can be combined with Radix Bupleuri (*Chai Hu*), Radix Albus Paeoniae Lactiflorae (*Bai Shao*), and Fructus Immaturus Citri Aurantii (*Zhi Shi*). For the treatment of diarrhea and dysentery tenesmus due to stomach and intestine damp heat, Bulbus Allii can be combined with Cortex Phellodendri (*Huang Bai*) and Cortex Fraxini (*Qin Pi*).

Dosage: 5-10g

Method of use: Decoct in water and administer internally.

Cautions & contraindications: This medicinal should not be administered to those with qi vacuity without stagnation or stomach weakness with torpid intake and no appetite.

Radix Linderae Strychnifoliae (*Wu Yao*)

Nature & flavor: Acrid and warm

Channel entry: Spleen, stomach, lungs, and kidneys

Functions: Normalizes the flow of qi and stops pain, warms the kidneys and scatters cold

Indications:

1. Used for stomach duct and abdominal distention and pain, vomiting, and diarrhea due to spleen-kidney dual vacuity, Radix Linderae Strychnifoliae can be combined with Fructus Evodiae Rutecarpae (*Wu Zhu Yu*) and Cortex Cinnamomi Cassiae (*Rou Gui*).

2. Used for urinary bladder vacuity chill with frequent urination and urinary incontinence, Radix Linderae Strychnifoliae can be combined with Fructus Alpiniae Oxyphyllae (*Yi Zhi Ren*).

3. Used for mounting pain and painful menstruation due to qi stagnation in the liver channel, Radix Linderae Strychnifoliae can be combined with Fructus Foeniculi Vulgaris (*Xiao Hui Xiang*), Semen Lichi Chinensis (*Li Zhi He*), and Semen Citri Reticulatae (*Ju He*).

Dosage: 6-10g

Method of use: Decoct in water and administer internally.

Pericarpium Citri Reticulatae Viride (*Qing Pi*)

Nature & flavor: Bitter, acrid, and warm

Channel entry: Liver and gallbladder

Functions: Courses the liver and breaks the qi, disperses accumulations and transforms stagnant food

Indications:

1. Used for chest and rib-side distention and pain, Pericarpium Citri Reticulatae Viride is commonly combined with Radix Bupleuri (*Chai Hu*) and Tuber Curcumae (*Yu Jin*). If there is accompanying blood stasis with enlargement of the liver or spleen, add Radix Salviae Miltiorrhizae (*Dan Shen*) and Carapax Amydae Sinensis (*Bie Jia*).

2. Used for breast distention and pain, this medicinal can be combined with Rhizoma Cyperi Rotundi (*Xiang Fu*) and Radix Bupleuri (*Chai Hu*). If there is breast abscess, Pericarpium Citri Reticulatae Viride can be combined with Squama Manitis Pentadactylis (*Chuan Shan Jia*), Semen Vaccariae Segetalis (*Wang Bu Liu Xing*), Flos Lonicerae Japonicae (*Jin Yin Hua*), and Herba Taraxaci Mongolici Cum Radice (*Pu Gong Ying*).

3. Used for food accumulation abdominal pain, Pericarpium Citri Reticulatae Viride can be combined with Fructus Crataegi (*Shan Zha*), Fructus Germinatus Hordei Vulgaris (*Mai Ya*), and Massa Medica Fermentata (*Shen Qu*).

Dosage: 3-10g

Method of use: Decoct in water and administer internally.

Cautions & contraindications: Because of this medicinal's harsh attacking nature, it should be used cautiously in those with qi vacuity.

Pericarpium Arecae Catechu (*Da Fu Pi*)

Nature & flavor: Acrid and slightly warm

Channel entry: Spleen, stomach, large intestine, and small intestine

Functions: Descends the qi and loosens the center, moves water and disperses swelling

Indications:

1. Used for damp obstruction and qi stagnation stomach duct and abdominal distention and oppression and uncrisp bowel movements, Pericarpium Arecae Catechu can be combined with Cortex Magnoliae Officinalis (*Hou Po*).

2. Used for water swelling, distention, and fullness, leg qi superficial edema, and inhibited urination, Pericarpium Arecae Catechu can be combined with Cortex Sclerotii Poriae Cocos (*Fu Ling Pi*) and Cortex Rhizomatis Zingiberis (*Jiang Pi*).

Dosage: 4.5-10g

Method of use: Decoct in water and administer internally.

Cautions & contraindications: Due to this medicinal's harsh attacking nature, it should be used cautiously in case of qi vacuity.

Fructus Meliae Toosendan (*Chuan Lian Zi*)

Nature & flavor: Bitter and cold. Has small toxins.

Channel entry: Liver, stomach, and small intestine

Functions: Soothes the liver, moves the qi, and stops pain, expels worms

Indications:

1. Used for chest, rib-side, stomach duct, and abdominal distention and pain due to liver depression qi stagnation, Fructus Meliae Toosendan is commonly combined with Rhizoma Corydalis Yanhusuo (*Yan Hu Suo*).

2. Used for mounting pain, Fructus Meliae Toosendan can be combined with Fructus Foeniculi Vulgaris (*Xiao Hui Xiang*).

3. Used for worm accumulation abdominal pain, Fructus Meliae Toosendan can be combined with Semen Arecae Catechu (*Bing Lang*) and Fructificatio Polypori Mylittae (*Lei Wan*).

Dosage: 5-10g

Method of use: Decoct in water and administer internally.

Cautions & contraindications: This medicinal is not appropriate for use in spleen-stomach vacuity cold.

Semen Litchi Chinensis (*Li Zhi He*)

Nature & flavor: Sweet, slightly bitter, and warm

Channel entry: Liver and kidneys

Functions: Moves the qi and scatters nodulations, dispels cold and stops pain

Indications:

1. Used for cold mounting abdominal pain, Semen Litchi Chinensis can be combined with Fructus Citri Aurantii (*Zhi Ke*).

2. Used for testicular swelling and pain, Semen Litchi Chinensis can be combined with Fructus Foeniculi Vulgaris (*Xiao Hui Xiang*).

Dosage: 6-10g

Method of use: Decoct in water and administer internally.

Cautions & contraindications: This medicinal should not be used without cold, damp, qi stagnation.

Lignum Aquilariae Agallochae (*Chen Xiang*)

Nature & flavor: Acrid, bitter, and slightly warm

Channel entry: Kidneys, spleen, and stomach

Functions: Moves the qi and stops pain, warms the center and stops vomiting

Indications:

1. Used for chest and abdominal distention, oppression, aching, and pain, stomach cold vomiting and hiccup, including nausea and vomiting during pregnancy, Lingum Aquilariae Agallochae can be combined with Folium Perillae Frutescentis (*Zi Su Ye*).

2. Used for kidney vacuity counterflow panting and rapid breathing, Lignum Aquilariae Agallochae can be combined with Semen Raphani Sativi (*Lai Fu Zi*).

Dosage: 1.5-4.5g

Method of use: Decoct in water and administer internally or taken in powders and pills. When decocted, add later. Some sources say this medicinal should not be decocted.

Cautions & contraindications: Use cautiously in those with central qi downward fall and those with yin vacuity with heat symptoms.

Lignum Santali Albi (*Tan Xiang*)

Nature & flavor: Acrid and warm

Channel entry: Spleen, stomach, and lungs

Functions: Moves the heart and warms the center, opens the stomach and stops pain

Indications:

1. Used for cold coagulation qi stagnation chest pain, Lingum Santali Albi can be combined with Radix Salviae Miltiorrhizae (*Dan Shen*).

2. Used for stomach pain and scanty eating, Lignum Santali Albi can be combined with Fructus Amomi (*Sha Ren*), Flos Caryophylli (*Ding Xiang*), and Herba Agastachis Seu Pogostemi (*Huo Xiang*).

Dosage: 1-3g

Method of use: Decoct in water and administer internally.

Cautions & contraindications: Due to this medicinal's windy, aromatic nature, it is contraindicated in those with yin vacuity with heat symptoms.

Fructus Citri Sacrodactylis (*Fo Shou*)

Nature & flavor: Acrid, bitter, sour, and warm

Channel entry: Liver, stomach, and spleen

Functions: Soothes the liver and rectifies the qi, harmonizes the stomach and stops pain

Indications:

1. Used for liver-stomach qi stagnation chest and rib-side distention and pain, and stomach duct glomus and fullness, Fructus Citri Sacrodactylis is commonly combined with Radix Auklandiae Lappae (*Mu Xiang*) and Pericarpium Citri Reticulatae Viride (*Qing Pi*).

2. Used for indigestion, devitalized eating and drinking, burping and belching, and vomiting and spitting, this medicinal can be combined with Fructus Amomi (*Sha Ren*), Fructus Cardamomi (*Bai Dou Kou*), and Rhizoma Pinelliae Ternatae (*Ban Xia*).

Dosage: 6-10g

Method of use: Decoct in water and administer internally.

Calyx Diospyros Khaki (*Shi Di*)

Nature & flavor: Bitter, astringent, and level

Channel entry: Lungs and stomach

Functions: Downbears counterflow and descends the qi

Indications: Used for hiccups, burping, or vomiting, chest and stomach duct glomus and fullness due to spleen-stomach vacuity cold, Calyx Diospyros Khaki is commonly combined with Flos Caryophylli (*Ding Xiang*) as in *Ding Xiang Shi Di Tang* (Clove & Persimmon Calyx Decoction).

Dosage: 4.5-10g

Method of use: Decoct in water and administer internally.

Semen Citri Reticulatae (*Ju He*)

Nature & flavor: Bitter and level

Channel entry: Liver

Functions: Rectifies the qi, scatters nodulations, and stops pain

Indications:

1. Used for lower abdominal mounting qi, testicular swelling and pain, and painful menstruation, Semen Citri Reticulatae can be combined with Fructus Foeniculi Vulgaris (*Xiao Hui Xiang*) and Radix Linderae Strychnifoliae (*Wu Yao*).

2. Used for the breast nodes, swelling, and pain, Semen Citri Reticulatae can be combined with Spica Prunellae Vulgaris (*Xia Ku Cao*), Radix Scrophulariae Ningpoensis (*Xuan Shen*), Bulbus Fritillariae Thunbergii (*Zhe Bei Mu*), and Concha Ostreae (*Mu Li*).

Dosage: 3-15g

Method of use: Decoct in water and administer internally.

8

Dispersing & abducting medicinals

Medicinals which mainly disperse food and abduct stagnation are called dispersing and abducting medicinals. This class of medicinals is able to disperse and eliminate food and drink accumulation and stagnation and restore the spleen and stomach's fortification and movement. Therefore, they are suitable for use in food accumulation non-transformation resulting in stomach duct and abdominal distention and fullness, burping, swallowing of acid, nausea and vomiting, and loss of constancy as well as spleen-stomach vacuity weakness indigestion.

Fructus Crataegi (*Shan Zha*)

Nature & flavor: Sour, sweet, and slightly warm

Channel entry: Spleen, stomach, and liver

Functions: Disperses food and transforms accumulations, quickens the blood and scatters stasis

Indications:

1. Used for food accumulation not transforming with symptoms of stomach duct and abdominal distention and fullness, no thought for food or drink, abdominal pain, and diarrhea. If there has been undisciplined eating and drinking or eating to much oily, slimy, meaty food and thus there is accumulation which is not dispersed, Fructus Crataegi can be used alone, decocted, and administered, or it can be combined with Massa Medica Fermentata (*Shen Qu*) and Fructus Germinatus Hordei Vulgaris (*Mai Ya*). If there is simultaneous stomach duct and abdominal distention and pain, Fructus Crataegi can be combined with Radix Auklandiae Lappae (*Mu Xiang*) and Fructus Citri Aurantii (*Zhi Ke*). For the treatment of food damage diarrhea and dysentry, Fructus Crataegi can be used stir-fried till scorched and then powdered. This is then administered mixed with warm water.

2. Used for postpartum stasis obstructing the abdomen pain and a lochia that will not cease, Fructus Crataegi can be used alone decocted in water with brown sugar added or it may be combined with Radix Angelicae Sinensis (*Dang Gui*), Radix Ligustici Wallichii (*Chuan Xiong*), Herba Leonuri Heterophylli (*Yi Mu Cao*), and Rhizoma Corydalis Yanhusuo (*Yan Hu Suo*).

In addition, Fructus Crataegi can be combined with Semen Cassiae Torae (*Jue Ming Zi*) for the treatment of hypertension and high cholesterol. These are boiled in water, white sugar is added, and this is drunk as a beverage tea. If Fructus Crataegi is combined with Flos Carthami Tinctorii (*Hong Hua*), Radix Salviae Miltiorrhizae (*Dan Shen*), and Radix Rubrus Paeoniae Lactiflorae (*Chi Shao*), it can be used for the treatment of angina pectoris and coronary heart disease.

Dosage: 10-15g and in larger doses up to 30-60g

Method of use: Decoct in water and administer internally. For dispersing food and transforming stasis, mostly use stir-fried. For stopping dysentery and transforming stasis, mostly use stir-fried till carbonized. For downbearing the blood pressure and cholesterol or for out-thrusting rashes, use uncooked.

Endothelium Corneum Gigeriae Galli (*Ji Nei Jin*)

Nature & flavor: Sweet, astringent, and level

Channel entry: Spleen, stomach, small intestine, and urinary bladder

Functions: Moves the spleen and disperses food, secures the essence and stops emission, transforms hardness and disperses stones

Indications:

1. Used for food accumulation not transforming, stomach duct and abdominal distention and fullness, no thought for food or drink, and children's gan accumulation, Endothelium Corneum Gigeriae Galli may be used alone, ground into powder, and taken or it may be combined with Fructus Crataegi (*Shan Zha*), Massa Medica Fermentata (*Shen Qu*), and Fructus Germinatus Hordei Vulgaris (*Mai Ya*). For those with fatigue, lack of strength, and other such symptoms of spleen vacuity, Endothelium Corneum Gigeriae Galli can be combined with Rhizoma Atractylodis Macrocephalae (*Bai Zhu*), Radix Dioscoreae Oppositae (*Shan Yao*), and Sclerotium Poriae Cocos (*Fu Ling*).

2. Used for enuresis and seminal emission. For the former, Endothelium Corneum Gigeriae Galli is commonly combined with Ootheca Mantidis (*Sang Piao Xiao*) and Fructus Rubi Chingii (*Fu Pen Zi*). For the latter, it can be combined with Semen Nelumbinis Nuciferae (*Lian Zi*) and Semen Cuscutae Chinensis (*Tu Si Zi*).

3. Used for bound stone conditions. For the treatment of liver-gallbladder bound stones, Endothelium Corneum Gigeriae Galli is commonly combined with Herba Lysimachiae (*Jin Qian Cao*) and Tuber Curcumae (*Yu Jin*). For the treatment of kidney and urinary bladder

bound stones, it is commonly combined with Semen Juglandis Regiae (*Hu Tao Ren*), Sporae Lygodii (*Hai Jin Sha*), and Herba Lysimachiae (*Jin Qian Cao*).

Dosage: 3-10g

Method of use: Decoct in water and administer internally. However, when ground into powder and washed down, 1.5-3g each time, its therapeutic effect is better than when decocted. Decocting this medicinal can easily decrease its effect.

Fructus Germinatus Hordei Vulgaris (*Mai Ya*)

Nature & flavor: Sweet and level

Channel entry: Spleen, stomach, and liver

Functions: Disperses food, returns the breast milk, *i.e.*, stops lactation

Indications:

1. Used for food accumulation not transforming, no thought of food or drink, and stomach duct oppression and abdominal distention, Fructus Germinatus Hordei Vulgaris is commonly combined with Fructus Crataegi (*Shan Zha*) and Massa Medica Fermentata (*Shen Qu*).

2. Used for stopping women's lactation or if the breast milk is depressed and accumulating with breast distention and pain, Fructus Germinatus Hordei Vulgaris can be used half uncooked and half stir-fried, decocted in water, and administered.

In addition, this ingredient also has the power to course the liver. Therefore, it can be used as an adjuvant medicinal for the treatment of liver depression qi stagnation conditions.

Dosage: 10-15g. However, when used alone for returning the breast milk, *i.e.*, stemming lactation, one may use as much as 60-120g.

Method of use: Decoct in water and administer internally. For dispersing food, one should use stir-fried. Otherwise, use uncooked.

Cautions & contraindications: This medicinal should not be used in women while breast-feeding.

Semen Raphani Sativi (*Lai Fu Zi*)

Nature & flavor: Acrid, sweet, and level

Channel entry: Spleen, stomach, and lungs

Functions: Disperses food and transforms accumulations, downbears the qi and transforms phlegm

Indications:

1. Used for food accumulation qi stagnation, stomach duct and abdominal distention and fullness, putrid eructations, and swallowing acid or abdominal pain and diarrhea or diarrhea which is not easily flowing, Semen Raphani Sativi is commonly combined with Fructus Crataegi (*Shan Zha*), Massa Medica Fermentata (*Shen Qu*), and Pericarpium Citri Reticulatae (*Chen Pi*) as in *Bao He Wan* (Protect Harmony Pills).

2. Used for phlegm drool blockage and exuberance, qi panting, and cough, Semen Raphani Sativi is commonly combined with Semen Sinapis Albae (*Bai Jie Zi*) and Fructus Perillae Frutescentis (*Zi Su Zi*) as in *San Zi Yang Qin Tang* (Three Seeds Nourish the Elderly Decoction).

Dosage: 3-10g

Method of use: Decoct in water and administer internally.

Cautions & contraindications: Due to this ingredient's ability to consume and cause detriment to the righteous qi, it should not be used in those with qi vacuity without food accumulation or phlegm stagnation.

Massa Medica Fermentata (*Shen Qu*)

Nature & flavor: Sweet, acrid, and warm

Channel entry: Spleen and stomach

Functions: Disperses food and transforms accumulations, abducts stagnation and harmonizes the stomach

Indications: Used for food stagnation, primarily of cereals, resulting in stomach duct and abdominal distention and fullness, scanty eating, and diarrhea. For the treatment of spleen vacuity diarrhea with accompanying food stagnation, Massa Medica Fermentata can be combined with Rhizoma Atractylodis Macrocephalae (*Bai Zhu*). For food accumulation and qi stagnation, Massa Medica Fermentata can be combined with Fructus Citri Aurantii (*Zhi Ke*). For pediatric gan condition due to food stagnation, this medicinal can be combined with Semen Arecae Catechu (*Bing Lang*). And for abdominal pain due to food stagnation, it can be combined with Radix Auklandiae Lappae (*Mu Xiang*) and Fructus Amomi (*Sha Ren*).

Dosage: 6-15g

Method of use: Decoct in water and administer internally. For harmonizing the stomach and dispersing food, mostly use stir-fried. For stopping diarrhea and dysentery, mostly use stir-fried till scorched.

9

Worm-expelling medicinals

Medicinals which mainly have the action of expelling and eliminating or killing and dousing parasites are called worm-expelling medicinals. This type of medicinal is mainly used for intestinal parasites, such as roundworms, enterobiasis, tapeworms, and pinworms.

When using worm-expelling medicinals, one should pay attention to the following points: One should take these medicinals on an empty stomach so that they have an easier, *i.e.*, better, action on the worm bodies. Some of these medicinals have toxins. Therefore one must pay attention to their dosage. If there is fever or if abdominal pain is relatively severe, one should temporarily suspend their use. These medicinals should be used cautiously in pregnant women and those who are old and weak.

Fructus Quisqualis Indicae (*Shi Jun Zi*)

Nature & flavor: Sweet and warm

Channel entry: Spleen and stomach

Functions: Kills worms and disperses accumulations

Indications:

1. Used for roundworm disease and enterobiasis, Fructus Quisqualis Indicae can be used alone, stir-fried till aromatic, chewed and eaten, or it can be combined with Cortex Radicis Meliae Azardachis (*Ku Lian Pi*) and Semen Arecae Catechu (*Bing Lang*).

2. Used for pediatric gan accumulation with bodily emaciation, an enlarged abdomen, and a sallow yellow facial complexion, Fructus Quisqualis Indicae is commonly combined with Radix Codonopsitis Pilosulae (*Dang Shen*), Rhizoma Atractylodis Macrocephalae (*Bai Zhu*), Endothelium Corneum Gigeriae Galli (*Ji Nei Jin*), and Semen Arecae Catechu (*Bing Lang*).

Dosage: 6-12g. If stir-fried and chewed, take 10-20 grains each time. Children should take 1-1.5 grains each day for each year of age, but not exceeding a total of 20 grains.

Method of use: Decoct in water and administer internally.

Cautions & contraindications: If this medicinal is taken in large amounts with food or tea, it may lead to the arising of the side effects of hiccup, dizziness, and vomiting and spitting. Typically, these will spontaneously relax and resolve after stopping the medicinal. If necessary, one can use whatever other medicinals are indicated by the condition. When taking this medicinal, drinking strong tea is contraindicated.

Semen Arecae Catechu (*Bing Lang*)

Nature & flavor: Bitter, acrid, and warm

Channel entry: Stomach and large intestine

Functions: Kills worms and disperses accumulations, descends the qi and frees the flow of the stool, disinhibits water and disperses swelling

Indications:

1. Used for many types of intestinal tract parasitoses. For cestodiasis and fasciolopsiasis, Semen Arecae Catechu can be used alone, decocted, and administered. If combined with Semen Cucurbitae (*Nan Gua Zi*), its effect of expelling and killing worms is able to be increased and strengthened. For roundworms or pinworms, it can be combined with Cortex Radicis Meliae Azardachis (*Ku Lian Pi*) and Fructificatio Polypori Mylittae (*Lei Wan*). For enterobiasis, it can be combined with Radix Stemonae (*Bai Bu*).

2. Used for food accumulation qi stagnation with abdominal distention and constipation or diarrhea and dysentery with tenesmus, Semen Arecae Catechu is commonly combined with Radix Auklandiae Lappae (*Mu Xiang*) and Radix Et Rhizoma Rhei (*Da Huang*) as in *Mu Xiang Bing Lang Wan* (Auklandia & Areca Pills) and *Shao Yao Tang* (Peony Decoction).

3. Used for leg qi swelling and pain and water swelling repletion patterns. For the former, Semen Arecae Catechu is commonly combined with Fructus Chaenomelis Lagenariae (*Mu Gua*), Fructus Evodiae Rutecarpae (*Wu Zhu Yu*), and Folium Perillae Frutescentis (*Zi Su Ye*) as in *Ji Ming San* (Cock Crow Powder). For the latter, it can be combined with Radix Phytolaccae (*Shang Lu*), Cortex Sclerotii Poriae Cocos (*Fu Ling Pi*), and Rhizoma Alismatis (*Ze Xie*) as in *Shu Zao Yin Zi* (Course & Chisel Drink).

Dosage: 6-15g. When used alone to treat cestodiasis and fasciolopsiasis, the dosage may be as much as 60-120g.

Method of use: Decoct in water and administer internally

134

Cautions & contraindications: This medicinal should not be used for those with spleen vacuity loose stools.

Semen Cucurbitae (*Nan Gua Zi*)

Nature & flavor: Sweet and level

Channel entry: Stomach and large intestine

Functions: Kills worms

Indications: Used for cestodiasis and roundworm disease. For the treatment of cestodiasis, Semen Cucurbitae is commonly combined with Semen Arecae Catechu (*Bing Lang*). In that case, 60-120g of Semen Cucurbitae is taken first. Then two hours later, 60-120g of Semen Arecae Catechu is decocted and taken. Another half hour later, 15g of Mirabilitum (*Mang Xiao*) is mixed with water and taken in order to promote the expulsion and discharge of the worms. For the treatment of roundworms, Semen Cucurbitae can be combined with Fructus Quisqualis Indice (*Shi Jun Zi*), Fructus Pruni Mume (*Wu Mei*), and Cortex Radicis Meliae Azardachis (*Ku Lian Pi*).

In addition, prolonged administration of large doses of this medicinal can also be used for the treatment of schistosomiasis.

Dosage: 60-120g

Method of use: Either the husked or unhusked seed should be ground into fine powder. This should be mixed with chilled boiled water and administered. It is also ok to swallow after chewing and macerating.

10

Stop bleeding medicinals

Medicinals which mainly control and stop internal and external bleeding are called stop bleeding medicinals. This group of medicinals is divided into cooling the blood and stop bleeding medicinals, restraining, constraining, and stop bleeding medicinals, transforming stasis stop bleeding medicinals, and warming the channels stop bleeding medicinals. Each of the above has their own use, however, as a group, these medicinals are suitable for use in hemorrhagic diseases, such as spitting of blood, hacking of blood, spontaneous ejection of blood, hematuria, hemafecia, flooding and leaking, purpura, and bleeding due to external injury.

When using stop bleeding medicinals, it is important to prevent retention of static blood. If there are signs and symptoms of static blood, it is not appropriate to use cooling the blood or restraining and constraining stop bleeding medicinals alone.

Herba Cephalanoploris (*Xiao Ji*)

Nature & flavor: Sweet and cool

Channel entry: Heart and liver

Functions: Cools the blood and stops bleeding, resolves toxins and disperses welling abscesses

Indications:

1. Used for blood heat frenetic movement resulting in hacking blood, *i.e.*, hemoptysis, spontaneous ejection of blood, *i.e.*, epistaxis, spitting of blood, *i.e.*, hematemesis, hematuria, and flooding and leaking, Herba Cephalanoploris is especially effective for hematuria. It is commonly combined with Pollen Typhae (*Pu Huang*), Caulis Akebiae (*Mu Tong*), and Talcum (*Hua Shi*) as in *Xiao Ji Yin Zi* (Cephalanoplos Drink).

2. Used for heat toxin sores and welling abscesses, Herba Cephalanoploris can be used alone and taken internally or the fresh herb can be pounded and macerated and applied externally.

Dosage: 10-15g; fresh, use 30-60g

Method of use: Decoct in water and administer internally. Externally, use a suitable amount.

Radix Sanguisorbae (*Di Yu*)

Nature & flavor: Bitter, sour, astringent, and slightly cold

Channel entry: Liver, stomach, and large intestine

Functions: Cools the blood and stops bleeding, resolves toxins and constrains sores

Indications:

1. Used for various types of hemorrhagic conditions, Radix Sanguisorbae is especially suitable for lower burner blood heat resulting in hemafecia, hemorrhoidal bleeding, bloody dysentery, and flooding and leaking. For the treatment of hemafecia and hemorrhoidal bleeding, Radix Sanguisorbae is commonly combined with Flos Immaturus Sophorae Japonicae (*Huai Hua*). For the treatment of blood heat flooding and leaking, it can be combined with uncooked Radix Rehmanniae (*Sheng Di*) and Radix Scutellariae Baicalensis (*Huang Qin*). For the treatment of bloody dysentery, it can be combined with Rhizoma Coptidis Chinensis (*Huang Lian*) and Radix Auklandiae Lappae (*Mu Xiang*).

2. Used for scalds, eczema, and skin ulcers. For the treatment of scalds, Radix Sanguisorbae can be used alone ground into powder, mixed with sesame oil, and applied. Or it may be combined with powdered Cortex Phellodendri (*Huang Bai*), uncooked Gypsum Fibrosum (*Shi Gao*), Radix Et Rhizoma Rhei (*Da Huang*), and Calcitum (*Han Shui Shi*) at a ratio of 8:4:4:2:2, mixed with sesame oil, and applied. For the treatment of eczema and skin ulcers, cotton gauze can be soaked in a thick decoction made from uncooked Radix Sanguisorbae and applied externally, or Radix Sanguisorbae may be combined with calcined Gypsum Fibrosum (*Shi Gao*) and Alum (*Ku Fan*), ground into fine powder, and spread on the affected area.

Dosage: 10-30g. Externally, use a suitable amount.

Method of use: Decoct in water and administer internally. For resolving toxins and constraining sores, mostly use uncooked. For stopping bleeding, one can use stir-fried till carbonized.

Cautions & contraindications: For large burn areas, it is not appropriate to use Radix Sanguisorbae preparations applied externally in order to prevent hepatitis due to poisoning from the absorption of hydrolytic tannins.

Rhizoma Bletillae Striatae (*Bai Ji*)

Nature & flavor: Bitter, sweet, astringent, and slightly cold

Channel entry: Lungs, liver, and stomach

Functions: Restrains, constrains, and stops bleeding, disperses swelling and engenders muscle, *i.e.*, flesh

Indications:

1. Used for hacking of blood, spitting of blood, and external injury bleeding, especially bleeding from the lung and stomach, Rhizoma Bletillae Striatae can be used alone ground into powder and taken in glutinous rice soup or mixed with cool blooded water. It may also be combined with Radix Pseudoginseng (*San Qi*) and taken in powder form. For the treatment of taxation cough hacking of blood, *i.e.*, hemoptysis due to pulmonary tuberculosis, Rhizoma Bletillae Striatae can be combined with Folium Eriobotryae Japonicae (*Pi Pa Ye*), powdered Gecko (*Ge Jie*), and Gelatinum Corii Asini (*E Jiao*). For hematemesis accompanied by stomach pain and acid regurgitation, it can be combined with Os Sepiae Seu Sepiellae (*Wu Zei Gu*) as in *Wu Ji San* (Cuttle Bone & Bletilla Powder). For the treatment of external injury bleeding, Rhizoma Bletillae Striatae can be ground into powder and applied externally.

2. Used for sore and welling abscess swelling and toxins. In the initial stage when the sore has not ruptured, Rhizoma Bletillae Striatae is commonly combined with Flos Lonicerae Japonicae (*Jin Yin Hua*), Radix Trichosanthis Kirlowii (*Tian Hua Fen*), and Spina Gleditschiae Chinensis (*Zao Jiao Ci*). If the sore has ruptured but its mouth does not close for a long time, Rhizoma Bletillae Striatae can be ground into powder and applied externally.

In addition, when this ingredient is ground into powder and mixed into an ointment with sesame oil, it can be used to treat cracking of the hands and feet, anal fissures, and scalds.

Dosage: 3-10g. When ground into powder, take 1-3g each time. Externally, use a suitable amount.

Method of use: Decoct in water and administer internally.

Cautions & contraindications: Opposes or reverses Radix Aconiti (*Wu Tou*).

Rhizoma Imperatae Cylindricae (*Bai Mao Gen*)

Nature & flavor: Sweet and cold

Channel entry: Lungs, stomach, small intestine, and urinary bladder

Functions: Cools the blood and stops bleeding, clears heat and disinhibits urination

Indications:

1. Used for blood heat spitting of blood, spontaneous ejection of blood, and hematuria, Rhizoma Imperatae Cylindricae is commonly combined with uncooked Radix Rehmanniae (*Sheng Di*) and Nodus Rhizomatis Nelumbinis Nuciferae (*Ou Jie*).

2. Used for heat disease vexatious thirst, Rhizoma Imperatae Cylindricae is commonly combined with Rhizoma Phragmitis Communis (*Lu Gen*).

3. Used for jaundice, water swelling, and heat strangury, astringency, and pain, Rhizoma Imperatae Cylindricae can be combined with Semen Phaseoli Calcarati (*Chi Xiao Dou*).

Dosage: 10-30g or 30-60g when used fresh (The fresh ingredient is better.)

Method of use: Decoct in water and administer internally.

Radix Pseudoginseng (*San Qi*)

Nature & flavor: Sweet, slightly bitter, and warm

Channel entry: Liver and stomach

Functions: Transforms stasis and stops bleeding, quickens the blood and stabilizes pain

Indications:

1. Used internally and externally for various types of hemorrhagic conditions, Radix Pseudoginseng is especially suitable when bleeding is accompanied by stasis and stagnation. Used alone, Radix Pseudoginseng can be taken by swallowing its powder, or it can be combined with Ophicalcitum (*Hua Rui Shi*) and Crinis Carbonisatus (*Xue Yu Tan*).

2. Used for detriment and damage due to fall and strike, stasis, swelling, aching, and pain, Radix Pseudoginseng can be both taken internally and applied externally. It may be used

alone or can be combined with Resina Olibani (*Ru Xiang*), Resina Myrrhae (*Mo Yao*), and Eupolyphaga Seu Ophistoplatia (*Zhe Chong*).

In addition, in recent years, Radix Pseudoginseng has been shown to have a definite therapeutic effect in the treatment of angina pectoris due to coronary heart disease.

Dosage: 1-3g. Externally, use a suitable amount.

Method of use: Grind into fine powder and swallow to take.

Cautions & contraindications: Because its nature is warm, for bleeding with simultaneous yin vacuity oral dryness, this medicinal should be used in combination with yin-enriching, blood-cooling medicinals.

Pollen Typhae (*Pu Huang*)

Nature & flavor: Sweet and level

Channel entry: Liver and pericardium

Functions: Stops bleeding, transforms stasis

Indications:

1. Used for hacking of blood, spontaneous ejection of blood, spitting of blood, hematuria, hemafecia, flooding and leaking, and cutting injury bleeding of various types. Pollen Typhae can be powdered and used alone or it can be combined with Herba Agrimoniae Pilosae (*Xian He Cao*), Herba Ecliptae Prostratae (*Han Lian Cao*), and Cacumen Biotae Orientalis (*Ce Bai Ye*). For the treatment of external injury bleeding, it can be used alone applied externally.

2. Used for heart and abdominal aching and pain, postpartum abdominal pain, and menstrual movement abdominal pain categorized as static blood internally obstructing, Pollen Typhae is commonly combined with Feces Trogopterori Seu Pteromi (*Wu Ling Zhi*) as in *Shi Xiao San* (Loose a Smile Powder).

In addition, this ingredient simultaneously has some power to disinhibit urination. It is commonly used for bloody strangury, astringency, and pain, for which it is combined with Semen Abutilonis Seu Malvae (*Dong Kui Zi*) and uncooked Radix Rehmanniae (*Sheng Di*) as in *Pu Huang San* (Pollen Typhae Powder).

Dosage: 5-10g. Three grams may be washed down each time. Externally, use a suitable amount.

Method of use: Decoct in water and administer internally. It should be wrapped during decoction. The uncooked is used to stop bleeding and is simultaneously able to move the blood and transform stasis. The stir-fried till carbonized is used to restrain, constrain, and stop bleeding.

Cautions & contraindications: Uncooked Pollen Typhae is able to cause contractions in the uterus. Therefore, it is contraindicated in pregnant women.

Folium Artemisiae Argyii (*Ai Ye*)

Nature & flavor: Bitter, acrid, and warm

Channel entry: Liver, spleen, and kidneys

Functions: Warms the channels and stops bleeding, scatters cold and stops pain

Indications:

1. Used for lower burner vacuity cold resulting in excessively profuse menstruation, flooding and leaking precipitation of blood, and fetal leakage precipitation of blood, Folium Artemisiae Argyii is commonly combined with Gelatinum Corii Asini (*E Jiao*), Radix Angelicae Sinensis (*Dang Gui*), and Radix Albus Paeoniae Lactiflorae (*Bai Shao*) as in *Jiao Ai Tang* (Donkey Skin Glue & Mugwort Decoction). The fresh herb can be combined with fresh uncooked Radix Rehmanniae (*Sheng Di*), fresh Folium Nelumbinis Nuciferae (*Ou Ye*), and fresh Cacumen Biotae Orientalis (*Ce Bai Ye*) for the treatment of blood heat frenetic movement spontaneous ejection of blood and spitting of blood as in *Si Sheng Wan* (Four Uncooked [Ingredients] Pills).

2. Used for lower burner vacuity cold menstrual irregularity, painful menstruation, abnormal vaginal discharge, lower abdominal chilly pain, and chilled uterus infertility, Folium Artemisiae Argyii is commonly combined with Rhizoma Cyperi Rotundi (*Xiang Fu*), Cortex Cinnamomi Cassiae (*Rou Gui*), and Fructus Evodiae Rutecarpae (*Wu Zhu Yu*) as in *Ai Fu Nuan Gong Wan* (Mugwort & Cyperus Warm the Palace Pills).

In addition, when this ingredient is decocted, it may be used externally as a wash for eczema and itching. Moxibustion of acupoints using Folium Artemisiae Argyii has the effect of warming and freeing the flow of the qi and blood, thrusting and extending the channels and network vessels, *i.e.*, promoting the circulation of the channels and network vessels,

Dosage: 3-10g. Externally, use a suitable amount.

Method of use: Decoct in water and administer internally. For warming the channels and stopping bleeding, one should use stir-fried. Otherwise use uncooked.

Cautions & contraindications: This medicinal should not be used alone in cases of yin vacuity blood heat.

Herba Agrimoniae Pilosae (*Xian He Cao*)

Nature & flavor: Bitter, astringent, and level

Channel entry: Lungs, liver, and spleen

Functions: Restrains, constrains, and stops bleeding, cures malaria, stops dysentery, and resolves toxins

Indications:

1. Used for various types of bleeding, primarily due to qi vacuity not managing, *i.e.*, not containing, the blood, Herba Agrimoniae Pilosae is commonly combined with Radix Astragali Membranacei (*Huang Qi*). In addition, for the treatment of women's flooding and leaking or dark colored hemafecia, Herba Agrimoniae Pilosae can be combined with Os Sepiae Seu Sepiellae (*Wu Zei Gu*). For hematuria, Herba Agrimoniae Pilosae can be combined with Rhizoma Imperatae Cyclindricae (*Bai Mao Gen*). And for hacking of blood due to lung yin vacuity with vacuity heat damaging the network vessels, Herba Agrimoniae Pilosae can be combined with Gelatinum Corii Asini (*E Jiao*).

2. For chronic diarrhea and dysentery, this medicinal can be combined with Flos Hibisci (*Mu Jin Hua*).

3. For killing "worms" causing hemophilus vaginal tract inflammation resulting in genital area itching, this medicinal can be used as a vaginal douche.

Dosage: 10-15g. In larger does, this medicinal can be used up to 30-60g. Externally, use a suitable amount.

Method of use: Decoct in water and administer internally.

Flos Immaturus Sophorae Japonicae (*Huai Hua Mi*)

Nature & flavor: Bitter and slightly cold

Channel entry: Liver and large intestine

Functions: Cools the blood and stops bleeding, clears the liver and drains fire

Indications:

1. Used for bleeding hemorrhoids, hemafecia, and bloody dysentery due to heat forcing the blood to move frenetically outside its pathways, Fructus Immaturus Sophorae Japonicae is commonly combined with Cacumen Biotae Orientalis (*Ce Bai Ye*) and carbonized Herba Seu Flos Schizonepetae Tenuifoliae (*Jing Jie Sui*).

2. Used for liver heat red eyes, headache, dizziness, vertigo, and insomnia, Flos Immaturus Sophorae Japonicae is commonly combined with Herba Siegesbeckiae (*Xi Xian Cao*) or with Rhizoma Coptidis Chinensis (*Huang Lian*).

Dosage: 4.5-10g

Method of use: Decoct in water and administer internally.

Radix Rubiae Cordifoliae (*Qian Cao Gen*)

Nature & flavor: Bitter and cold

Channel entry: Heart and liver

Functions: Cools the blood, stops bleeding, dispels stasis, and frees the flow of the channels (or menses)

Indications:

1. Used for various types of hemorrhagic conditions due to blood heat. For the treatment of bloody dysentery, Radix Rubiae Cordifoliae can be combined with Cortex Phellodendri (*Huang Bai*) and Rhizoma Coptidis Chinensis (*Huang Lian*). For the treatment of spitting of blood and spontaneous ejection of blood, Radix Rubiae Cordifoliae can be combined with uncooked Radix Rehmanniae (*Sheng Di*) and Rhizoma Bletillae Striatae (*Bai Ji*). For women's flooding and leaking, Radix Rubiae Cordifoliae can be combined with Cacumen Biotae Orientalis (*Ce Bai Ye*) and Radix Sanguisorbae (*Di Yu*). For allergic purpura, this

medicinal can be combined with Radix Lithospermi Seu Arnebiae (*Zi Cao*) and Radix Salviae Miltiorrhizae (*Dan Shen*).

2. Used for stasis heat painful menstruation or blocked menstruation, Radix Rubiae Cordifoliae is commonly combined with Radix Salviae Miltiorrhizae (*Dan Shen*) or with Flos Carthami Tinctorii (*Hong Hua*) and Radix Rubrus Paeoniae Lactiflorae (*Chi Shao*).

3. Used for joint and sinew impediment pain and swelling and pain due to fall and strike, Radix Rubiae Cordifoliae can be combined with Radix Rubrus Paeoniae Lactiflorae (*Chi Shao*) and Herba Lycopi Lucidi (*Ze Lan*).

Dosage: 6-10g

Method of use: Decoct in water and administer internally.

Cacumen Biotae Orientalis (*Ce Bai Ye*)

Nature & flavor: Bitter, astringent, and cold

Channel entry: Heart, liver, and large intestine

Functions: Cools the blood and stops bleeding, engenders muscle, *i.e.*, flesh, and blackens the hair

Indications:

1. Used for various types of hemorrhagic conditions. For spitting blood, hacking blood, or spontaneous ejection of blood due to heat, Cacumen Biotae Orientalis can be combined with uncooked Radix Rehmanniae (*Sheng Di*) and uncooked Nodus Rhizomatis Nelumbinis Nuciferae (*Ou Jie*). For women's flooding and leaking, Cacumen Biotae Orientalis can be combined with Pollen Typhae (*Pu Huang*). For vacuity cold bleeding, Cacumen Biotae Orientalis can be combined with Folium Artemisiae Argyii (*Ai Ye*) and dry Rhizoma Zingiberis (*Gan Jiang*).

2. Used for blackening the hair in young or middle-aged persons where there is blood heat blood vacuity and falling hair or premature greying of the hair, Cacumen Biotae Orientalis is commonly combined with Radix Polygoni Multiflori (*He Shou Wu*), Fructus Ligustri Lucidi (*Nu Zhen Zi*), and uncooked Radix Rehmanniae (*Sheng Di*).

In addition, used alone, Cacumen Biotae Orientalis can be applied externally to the initial stage of burns.

Dosage: 6-12g. Externally, use a suitable amount.

Method of use: Decoct in water and administer internally or powder, mix with sesame oil and lard, and apply externally to burns.

Nodus Rhizomatis Nelumbinis Nuciferae (*Ou Jie*)

Nature & flavor: Sweet, astringent, and level

Channel entry: Lungs, stomach, and liver

Functions: Stops bleeding, disperses stasis

Indications: Used for lung and/or stomach heat causing spitting of blood and hacking of blood. For the former, Nodus Rhizomatis Nelumbinis Nuciferae is commonly combined with Rhizoma Bletillae Striatae (*Bai Ji*) and Radix Rubiae Cordifoliae (*Qian Cao Gen*). For the latter, Nodus Rhizomatis Nelumbinis Nuciferae is often combined with uncooked Radix Rehmanniae (*Sheng Di*), Gelatinum Corii Asini (*E Jiao*), and Bulbus Fritillariae Cirrhosae (*Chuan Bei Mu*).

Dosage: 10-15g. When used fresh and in decoction, one can use up to 30-60g.

Method of use: Decoct in water and administer internally. For cooling the blood and transforming stasis, use uncooked. For constraining, astringing, and stopping bleeding, one should use stir-fried till carbonized.

Terra Flava Usta (*Fu Long Gan*)

Nature & flavor: Acrid and slightly warm

Channel entry: Spleen and stomach

Functions: Warms the blood and stops bleeding, warms the stomach and stops vomiting, stops diarrhea

Indications:

1. Used for enduring spleen qi vacuity bleeding, especially blood in the stool which is dark or blackish in color, Terra Flava Usta is often combined with Cortex Cinnamomi Cassiae (*Rou Gui*), Folium Artemisiae Argyii (*Ai Ye*), and Radix Angelicae Sinensis (*Dang Gui*).

2. Used for spleen vacuity nausea and vomiting during pregnancy, Terra Flava Usta can be combined with uncooked Rhizoma Zingiberis (*Sheng Jiang*), Rhizoma Pinelliae Ternatae (*Ban Xia*), and Pericarpium Citri Reticulatae (*Chen Pi*).

3. Used for spleen-stomach vacuity cold diarrhea and dysentery, Terra Flava Usta can be combined with Radix Codonopsitis Pilosulae (*Dang Shen*), Rhizoma Atractylodis Macrocephalae (*Bai Zhu*), and Sclerotium Poriae Cocos (*Fu Ling*).

In addition, this medicinal can be applied externally for the treatment of wet, weeping diaper rash.

Dosage: 15-60g. Externally, use a suitable amount.

Method of use: Decoct in water and administer internally. Wrap in a cotton bag during decoction. Externally, apply to the affected area as a dusting powder.

Petiolus Trachycarpi (*Zong Lu*)

Nature & flavor: Bitter, astringent, and level

Channel entry: Lungs, liver, and large intestine

Functions: Restrains, constrains, astringes, and stops bleeding

Indications: Used for spitting of blood, spontaneous ejection of blood, hematuria, hemafecia, and flooding and leaking of blood downward. For instance, for the treatment of women's flooding and leaking, Petiolus Trachycarpi is combined with Os Sepiae Seu Sepiellae (*Wu Zei Gu*), Radix Rubiae Cordifoliae (*Qian Cao Gen*), and Galla Rhois Chinensis (*Wu Bei Zi*) as in *Gu Chong Tang* (Secure the *Chong* Decoction).

Dosage: 3-10g

Method of use: Decoct in water and administer internally. Typically, this medicinal is used carbonized.

11

Blood-quickening, stasis-dispelling medicinals

Medicinals whose main effect is to free the flow of and disinhibit the blood vessels, promote the movement of the blood, and disperse and scatter static blood are called blood-quickening, stasis-dispelling medicinals or blood-quickening, stasis-transforming medicinals. Among these, those which have an even stronger action of quickening the blood and transforming stasis are called blood-breaking medicinals.

Blood-quickening, stasis-dispelling medicinals are mostly acrid, warm, moving, and scattering in nature. Because they free the flow of, extend, and quicken the blood's movement and disperse and scatter stasis and stagnation, they can be used to free the flow of the channels (or menses), disinhibit impediment, disperse swelling, and stop pain. They are suitable in various types of disease conditions where there is unsmooth movement of the blood of static blood obstructing internally, such as static blood blocked menstruation, painful menstruation, postpartum stasis obstruction abdominal pain, concretions, conglomerations, accumulations, and lumps, fall and strike detriment and damage, sore and welling abscess swelling and pain, and qi stagnation blood stasis resulting in chest, rib-side, stomach duct, and abdominal pain.

This category of medicinal is not appropriate in women's excessively profuse menstruation and it should be used cautiously or is contraindicated in pregnant women.

Radix Ligustici Wallichii (*Chuan Xiong*)

Nature & flavor: Acrid and warm

Channel entry: Liver, gallbladder, and pericardium

Functions: Quickens the blood and moves the qi, dispels wind and stops pain

Indications:

1. Used for qi stagnation blood stasis resulting in menstrual irregularity, painful menstruation, blocked menstruation, difficult birth, a postpartum lochia which does not descend, stasis obstruction abdominal pain, rib-side and flank pain, numbness, aching, and

pain of the extremities, detriment and damage due to fall and strike, and sore and welling abscess swelling and pain, Radix Ligustici Wallichii is always combined with Radix Angelicae Sinensis (*Dang Gui*). Then, depending on different diseases, these are combined with other medicinals. For instance, when used to regulate menstruation, it can be combined with Radix Rubrus Paeoniae Lactiflorae (*Chi Shao*) and Rhizoma Cyperi Rotundi (*Xiang Fu*). For difficult birth, it can be combined with Radix Achyranthis Bidentatae (*Niu Xi*) and Plastrum Testundinis (*Gui Ban*). For postpartum abdominal pain, it can be combined with Herba Leonuri Heterophylli (*Yi Mu Cao*) and Semen Pruni Persicae (*Tao Ren*). For rib-side pain, it can be combined with Radix Bupleuri (*Chai Hu*) and Rhizoma Cyperi Rotundi (*Xiang Fu*). For numbness of the extremities or pain due to injury from fall and strike, it can be combined with Radix Rubrus Paeoniae Lactiflorae (*Chi Shao*) and Flos Carthami Tinctorii (*Hong Hua*). And for sore and welling abscesses which have difficulty rupturing, one can combine Radix Ligustici Wallichii with Radix Astragali Membranacei (*Huang Qi*), Flos Lonicerae Japonicae (*Jin Yin Hua*), and Spina Gleditschiae Chinensis (*Zao Jiao Ci*)

2. Used for headache, wind damp impediment pain. For the treatment of wind cold headache, Radix Ligustici Wallichii can be combined with Radix Angelicae Dahuricae (*Bai Zhi*), Radix Ledebouriellae Divaricatae (*Fang Feng*), and Herba Asari Cum Radice (*Xi Xin*) as in *Chuan Xiong Cha Tiao San* (Ligusticum & Tea Mixed Powder). For the treatment of wind heat headache, Radix Ligustici Wallichii can be combined with Flos Chrysanthemi Morifolii (*Ju Hua*), Gyspum Fibrosum (*Shi Gao*), and Bombyx Batryticatus (*Jiang Can*) as in *Chuan Xiong San* (Ligusticum Powder). For the treatment of wind damp headache, Radix Ligustici Wallichii can be combined with Radix Et Rhizoma Notopterygii (*Qiang Huo*), Radix Et Rhizoma Ligustici Chinensis (*Gao Ben*), and Radix Ledebouriellae Divaricatae (*Fang Feng*) as in *Qiang Huo Sheng Shi Tang* (Notopterygium Overcome Dampness Decoction). For the treatment of blood stasis headache, it can be combined with Radix Rubrus Paeoniae Lactiflorae (*Chi Shao*), Flos Carthami Tinctorii (*Hong Hua*), Radix Salviae Miltiorrhizae (*Dan Shen*), Radix Angelicae Dahuricae (*Bai Zhi*). For the treatment of blood vacuity headache, Radix Ligustici Wallichii can be combined with Radix Angelicae Sinensis (*Dang Gui*), cooked Radix Rehmanniae (*Shu Di*), Radix Albus Paeoniae Lactiflorae (*Bai Shao*), and Flos Chrysanthemi Morifolii (*Ju Hua*). For the treatment of wind damp impediment pain, it can be combined with Radix Ledebouriellae Divaricatae (*Fang Feng*), Radix Angelicae Pubescentis (*Du Huo*), Radix Gentianae Macrophyllae (*Qin Jiao*), and Ramulus Loranthi Seu Visci (*Sang Ji Sheng*).

In addition, Radix Ligustici Wallichii has been used in recent years for the treatment of angina pectoris due to coronary heart disease and ischemic cerebrovascular disease.

Dosage: 3-10g

Method of use: Decoct in water, adding later, and administer internally.

Cautions & contraindications: This medicinal should not be used in those with yin vacuity and qi weakness, taxation heat profuse sweating, liver yang headache, or women with excessively profuse menstruation.

Radix Salviae Miltiorrhizae (*Dan Shen*)

Nature & flavor: Bitter and slightly cold

Channel entry: Heart, pericardium, and liver

Functions: Quickens the blood and dispels stasis, cools the blood and disperses welling abscesses, nourishes the blood and quiets the spirit

Indications:

1. Used for static blood obstruction and stagnation resulting in various types of diseases. Because the nature of Radix Salviae Miltiorrhizae tends to be cold or cool, it is particularly suitable for static blood conditions with simultaneous symptoms of blood heat. For the treatment of gynecological menstrual and gestational conditions, Radix Salviae Miltiorrhizae is commonly combined with Flos Carthami Tinctorii (*Hong Hua*), Semen Pruni Persicae (*Tao Ren*), and Herba Leonuri Heterophylli (*Yi Mu Cao*). For the treatment of static blood qi stagnation resulting in heart and abdominal pain and stomach duct aching and pain, Radix Salviae Miltiorrhizae can be combined with Lignum Santali Albi (*Tan Xiang*) and Fructus Amomi (*Sha Ren*) as in *Dan Shen Yin* (Salvia Drink). For the treatment of concretions and conglomerations, accumulations and gatherings, it can be combined with Rhizoma Sparganii (*San Leng*), Rhizoma Curcumae Zedoariae (*E Zhu*), and Carapax Amydae Sinensis (*Bie Jia*). For the treatment of detriment and damage due to fall and strike, stasis, swelling, aching, and pain, Radix Salviae Miltiorrhizae is commonly combined with Radix Angelicae Sinensis (*Dang Gui*), Flos Carthami Tinctorii (*Hong Hua*), and Radix Ligustici Wallichii (*Chuan Xiong*). And for the treatment of heat impediment joint redness, swelling, aching, and pain, Radix Salviae Miltiorrhizae should be combined with Caulis Lonicerae Japonicae (*Ren Dong Teng*), Radix Rubrus Paeoniae Lactiflorae (*Chi Shao*), Radix Gentianae Macrophyllae (*Qin Jiao*), and Ramulus Mori Albi (*Sang Zhi*).

2. Used for sore and welling abscess swelling and pain, Radix Salviae Miltiorrhizae is commonly combined with Flos Lonicerae Japonicae (*Jin Yin Hua*), Fructus Forsythiae Suspensae (*Lian Qiao*), Resina Olibani (*Ru Xiang*), and Resina Myrrhae (*Mo Yao*).

3. Used for heat damaging the constructive and yin with heart vexation and restlessness, Radix Salviae Miltiorrhizae is commonly combined with uncooked Radix Rehmanniae

(*Sheng Di*), Radix Scrophulariae Ningpoensis (*Xuan Shen*), and Folium Bambusae (*Zhu Ye*) as in *Qing Gong Tang* (Clear the Palace Decoction). For heart blood insufficiency heart palpitations, insomnia, and impaired memory, Radix Salviae Miltiorrhizae can be used alone made into an alcohol tincture for administration, or it may be combined with Caulis Polygoni Multiflori (*Ye Jiao Teng*).

In addition, in recent years, Radix Salviae Miltiorrhizae has been used for the treatment of liver and spleen enlargement, coronary heart disease, thromboangitis, and ectopic pregnancy with definite therapeutic effects.

Dosage: 10-15g. For the treatment of thromboangitis and heat impediment, one can use 30-60g.

Method of use: Decoct in water and administer internally. Stir-frying in alcohol can increase this medicinal's effects of quickening the blood and dispelling stasis.

Cautions & contraindications: Opposes or reverses Radix Et Rhizoma Veratri (*Li Lu*).

Herba Leonuri Heterophylli (*Yi Mu Cao*)

Nature & flavor: Acrid, slightly bitter, and slightly cold

Channel entry: Heart, liver, and urinary bladder

Functions: Quickens the blood and dispels stasis, disinhibits urination and disperses swelling

Indications:

1. Used for static blood internal obstruction resulting in menstrual irregularity, uneasiness or lack of smoothness in the menstrual movement, lower abdominal distention and pain, blocked menstruation, postpartum static blood obstruction abdominal pain, a lochia which does not cease, detriment and damage due to fall and strike with stasis, swelling, aching, and pain, Herba Leonuri Heterophylli can be used alone taken as a syrup prepared with granular sugar. This is called *Yi Mu Cao Gao* (Leonurus Syrup). It can also be used in combination with Radix Angelicae Sinensis (*Dang Gui*), Radix Ligustici Wallichii (*Chuan Xiong*), and Radix Rubrus Paeoniae Lactiflorae (*Chi Shao*).

2. Used for inhibited urination and water swelling, Herba Leonuri Heterophyllii can be used alone after being powdered, decocted, and administered. Or it may be combined with

Rhizoma Imperatae Cylindricae (*Bai Mao Gen*), Sclerotium Poriae Cocos (*Fu Ling*), and Rhizoma Atractylodis Macrocephalae (*Bai Zhu*).

In addition, because this ingredient also has the power to clear heat and resolve toxins, it can be used for sore and welling abscess swelling and pain as well as skin itching and rashes when used either externally or taken internally. In recent years, it has been commonly used for the treatment of acute and chronic nephritis water swelling and coronary heart disease angina pectoris categorized as static blood obstruction and stagnation.

Dosage: 10-15g. For disinhibiting urination and dispersing swelling, one can use up to 30-60g. Externally, use a suitable amount.

Method of use: Decoct in water and administer internally, adding later. The fresh herb can be cleaned and washed and then pounded and macerated for external application.

Cautions & contraindications: It is not appropriate to use this medicinal if there is blood vacuity and not stasis and stagnation.

Rhizoma Corydalis Yanhusuo (*Yan Hu Suo*)

Nature & flavor: Acrid, bitter, and warm

Channel entry: Heart, liver, and spleen

Functions: Quickens the blood, moves the qi, stops pain

Indications: Used for qi and blood coagulation and stagnation resulting in chest, rib-side, stomach duct, abdominal, and extremity aching and pain, Rhizoma Corydalis Yanhusuo can be used alone, ground into powder, and swallowed, or it can be combined with other suitable medicinals depending aching and pain in different areas. For stomach duct and abdominal aching and pain, Rhizoma Corydalis Yanhusuo can be combined with Fructus Meliae Toosendan (*Chuan Lian Zi*). For chest impediment aching and pain, it can be combined with Lignum Santali Albi (*Tan Xiang*). For mounting qi aching and pain, it can be combined with Fructus Foeniculi Vulgaris (*Xiao Hui Xiang*). For menstrual movement abdominal pain, Rhizoma Corydalis Yanhusuo can be combined with Radix Angelicae Sinensis (*Dang Gui*), Radix Ligustici Wallichii (*Chuan Xiong*), and Rhizoma Cyperi Rotundi (*Xiang Fu*). For limb aching and pain, it can be combined with Radix Angelicae Sinensis (*Dang Gui*), Ramulus Cinnamomi Cassiae (*Gui Zhi*), and Radix Rubrus Paeoniae Lactiflorae (*Chi Shao*). For damage and pain due to fall and strike, Rhizoma Corydalis Yanhusuo can be combined with Radix Angelicae Sinensis (*Dang Gui*), Resina Olibani

(*Ru Xiang*), and Resina Myrrhae (*Mo Yao*). In sum, Rhizoma Corydalis Yanhusuo can be used for any pain categorized as qi stagnation and blood stasis in the whole body, no matter whether above or below, internal or external.

Dosage: 6-15g. When ground into powder and taken, administer 1.5-3g each time mixed with warm boiled water or chased by a decocted prescription.

Method of use: Decoct in water and administer internally. Vinegar stir-frying can increase the strength of Rhizoma Corydalis Yanhusuo's pain-stopping effect.

Tuber Curcumae (*Yu Jin*)

Nature & flavor: Acrid, bitter, and cold

Channel entry: Heart, liver, and gallbladder

Functions: Quickens the blood and stops pain, moves the qi and resolves depression, cools the blood and clears the heart, disinhibits the gallbladder, recedes jaundice

Indications:

1. Used for liver qi depression and stagnation and blood stasis obstructing internally resulting in various types aching and pain and concretions, conglomerations, accumulations, and lumps. For the treatment of chest, rib-side, stomach duct, and abdominal distention and pain, Tuber Curcumae can be combined with Radix Salviae Miltiorrhizae (*Dan Shen*), Radix Bupleuri (*Chai Hu*), Rhizoma Cyperi Rotundi (*Xiang Fu*), and Fructus Citri Aurantii (*Zhi Ke*). For the treatment of women's menstrual movement abdominal pain and breast distention and pain, Tuber Curcumae can be combined with Radix Bupleuri (*Chai Hu*), Rhizoma Cyperi Rotundi (*Xiang Fu*), Radix Angelicae Sinensis (*Dang Gui*), and Radix Albus Paeoniae Lactiflorae (*Bai Shao*). For the treatment of hypochondral concretions and lumps, distention, fullness, aching, and pain, Tuber Curcumae can be combined with Radix Salviae Miltiorrhizae (*Dan Shen*), Caparapx Amydae Sinensis (*Bie Jia*), Herba Lycopi Lucidi (*Ze Lan*), and Pericarpium Citri Reticulatae Viride (*Qing Pi*).

2. Used for damp warm disease dampness, turbidity confounding the clear orifices resulting in chest and stomach duct glomus and oppression, lack of clarity of the spirit will, and for phlegm heat internally blocking resulting in vexation, agitation, depression, oppression, epilepsy, and fright mania. For the former, Tuber Curcumae is commonly combined with Rhizoma Acori Graminei (*Shi Chang Pu*), Fructus Gardeniae Jasminoidis (*Zhi Zi*), and Succus Bambusae (*Zhu Li*) as in *Chang Pu Yu Jin Tang* (Acorus & Curcuma

Decoction). For the latter, Tuber Curcumae is commonly combined with Alum (*Bai Fan*) as in *Bai Jin Wan* (White Gold Pills, or Alum & Curcuma Pills).

3. Used for blood heat mixed with stasis spitting of blood, spontaneous ejection of blood, hematuria, and women's shifted, *i.e.*, vicarious, menstruation, Tuber Curcumae can be combined with uncooked Radix Rehmanniae (*Sheng Di*), Cortex Radicis Moutan (*Dan Pi*), Fructus Gardeniae Jasminoidis (*Zhi Zi*), and Radix Achyranthis Bidentatae (*Niu Xi*).

4. Used for damp heat jaundice, Tuber Curcumae is commonly combined with Herba Artemisiae Capillaris (*Yin Chen Hao*) and Fructus Gardeniae Jasminoidis (*Zhi Zi*).

Dosage: 6-12g

Method of use: Decoct in water and administer internally.

Cautions & contraindications: Fears Flos Caryophylli (*Ding Xiang*).

Flos Carthami Tinctorii (*Hong Hua*)

Nature & flavor: Acrid and warm

Channel entry: Heart and liver

Functions: Quickens the blood and frees the flow of the channels, dispels stasis and stops pain

Indications:

1. Used for blood stasis blocked menstruation, painful menstruation, and postpartum stasis obstruction abdominal pain, Flos Carthami Tinctorii is commonly combined with Semen Pruni Persicae (*Tao Ren*), Radix Angelicae Sinensis (*Dang Gui*), and Radix Ligustici Wallichii (*Chuan Xiong*) as in *Tao Hong Si Wu Tang* (Persica & Carthamus Four Materials Decoction). For the treatment of concretions, conglomerations, accumulations, and lumps within the abdomen, Flos Carthami Tinctorii can be combined with Rhizoma Sparganii (*San Leng*), Rhizoma Curcumae Zedoariae (*E Zhu*), and Radix Salviae Miltiorrhizae (*Dan Shen*).

2. Used for various types of static blood aching and pain. For the treatment of chest impediment chest pain, Flos Carthami Tinctorii is commonly combined with Radix Salviae Miltiorrhizae (*Dan Shen*), Radix Rubrus Paeoniae Lactiflorae (*Chi Shao*), and Radix Ligustici Wallichii (*Chuan Xiong*). For the treatment of static blood rib-side pain, it can be combined with Resina Olibani (*Ru Xiang*), Resina Myrrhae (*Mo Yao*), and Semen Pruni

Persicae (*Tao Ren*). For the treatment of damage and pain due to fall and strike, it can be combined with Lignum Sappan (*Su Mu*), Sanguis Draconis (*Xue Jie*), and Secretio Moschi Moschiferi (*She Xiang*). And for the treatment of sore and welling abscess swelling and pain, Flos Carthami Tinctorii can be combined with Herba Taraxaci Mongolici Cum Radice (*Pu Gong Ying*), Fructus Forsythiae Suspensae (*Lian Qiao*), and Radix Rubrus Paeoniae Lactiflorae (*Chi Shao*).

Dosage: 3-10g. This medicinal can be used in slightly larger doses up 15g.

Method of use: Decoct in water and administer internally.

Cautions & contraindications: This medicinal should not be used in pregnant women or those with excessively profuse menstruation.

Semen Pruni Persicae (*Tao Ren*)

Nature & flavor: Bitter, sweet, and level

Channel entry: Heart, liver, lungs, and large intestine

Functions: Quickens the blood and dispels stasis, moistens the intestines and frees the flow of the stool

Indications:

1. Used for blood stasis blocked menstruation, painful menstruation, postpartum stasis obstruction abdominal pain, and concretions, conglomerations, accumulations, and gatherings, Semen Pruni Persicae is commonly combined with Flos Carthami Tinctorii (*Hong Hua*), Radix Angelicae Sinensis (*Dang Gui*), Radix Ligustici Wallichii (*Chuan Xiong*), and Radix Rubrus Paeoniae Lactiflorae (*Chi Shao*) as in *Tao Hong Si Wu Tang* (Persica & Carthamus Four Materials Decoction). For the treatment of detriment and damage due to fall and strike with stasis, swelling, aching and pain, it can be combined with Flos Carthami Tinctorii (*Hong Hua*), Radix Angelicae Sinensis (*Dang Gui*), Radix Et Rhizoma Rhei (*Da Huang*), and Squama Manitis Pentadactylis (*Chuan Shan Jia*) as in *Fu Yuan Huo Xue Tang* (Restore the Source & Quicken the Blood Decoction).

2. Used for the initial stage of lung and intestinal abscesses. For the former, Semen Pruni Persicae is commonly combined with Rhizoma Phragmitis Communis (*Lu Gen*), Semen Benincasae Hispidae (*Dong Gua Ren*), and Semen Coicis Lachryma-jobi (*Yi Yi Ren*) as in *Wei Jing Tang* (Phragmites Decoction). For the latter, Semen Pruni Persicae is commonly combined with Radix Et Rhizoma Rhei (*Da Huang*), Cortex Radicis Moutan (*Dan Pi*),

Semen Benincasae Hispidae (*Dong Gua Ren*), and Mirabilitum (*Mang Xiao*) as in *Da Huang Mu Dan Tang* (Rhubard & Moutan Decoction).

3. Used for intestinal dryness constipation, Semen Pruni Persicae is commonly combined with Semen Cannabis Sativae (*Huo Ma Ren*) and Semen Trichosanthis Kirlowii (*Gua Lou Ren*).

Dosage: 6-10g

Method of use: Crush before using and then decoct in water and administer internally.

Cautions & contraindications: This medicinal should not be used in pregnant women, those with excessively profuse menstruation, or those with blood withering blocked menstruation.

Radix Achyranthis Bidentatae (*Niu Xi*)

Nature & flavor: Bitter, sour, and level

Channel entry: Liver and kidneys

Functions: Quickens the blood and dispels stasis, supplements the liver and kidneys, strengthens the sinews and bones, disinhibits urination and frees the flow of strangury, leads the blood to move downward

Indications:

1. Used for static blood obstruction and stagnation resulting in menstrual irregularity, painful menstruation, blocked menstruation, difficult birth, non-descension of the placenta, postpartum stasis obstruction abdominal pain, and damage and pain due to fall and strike, Radix Achyranthis Bidentatae is commonly combined with Flos Carthami Tinctorii (*Hong Hua*), Semen Pruni Persicae (*Tao Ren*), Radix Angelicae Sinensis (*Dang Gui*), and Radix Ligustici Wallichii (*Chuan Xiong*).

2. Used for low back and knee soreness and pain and lower limb lack of strength due to liver-kidney vacuity detriment, Radix Achyranthis Bidentatae can be combined with Radix Angelicae Sinensis (*Dang Gui*), cooked Radix Rehmanniae (*Shu Di*), Plastrum Testudinis (*Gui Ban*), and Os Tigridis (*Hu Gu*)[6] as in *Hu Qian Wan* (Tiger Crouching Pills). If due

---

[6] Tiger bone comes from a severely endangered species and no part of the tiger should be used in the manufacture of medicine. One can substitute pig bone for this ingredient.

to damp heat pouring downward, Radix Achyranthis Bidentatae is commonly combined with Rhizoma Atractylodis (*Cang Zhu*), Cortex Phellodendri (*Huang Bai*), and Semen Coicis Lachryma-jobi (*Yi Yi Ren*) as in *Si Miao San* (Four Wonders Powder). If categorized as a wind damp impediment pattern, it is commonly combined with Radix Angelicae Pubescentis (*Du Huo*), Ramulus Loranthi Seu Visci (*Sang Ji Sheng*), and Cortex Eucommiae Ulmoidis (*Du Zhong*) as in *Du Huo Ji Sheng Tang* (Angelica Pubescens & Loranthus Decoction).

3. Used for hematuria, inhibited urination, and urinary tract astringency and pain, Radix Achyranthis Bidentatae can be combined with Radix Angelicae Sinensis (*Dang Gui*), Herba Dianthi (*Qu Mai*), Medulla Tetrapanacis Papyriferi (*Tong Cao*), and Talcum (*Hua Shi*) as in *Niu Xi Tang* (Achyranthes Decoction).

4. Used for spitting blood, spontaneous ejection of blood, bleeding teeth, *i.e.*, gums, sores in the mouth and on the tongue, and headache and dizziness. For the treatment of static blood spitting and spontaneous ejection of blood, Radix Achyranthis Bidentatae can be combined with Rhizoma Imperatae Cylindricae (*Bai Mao Gen*), Fructus Gardeniae Jasminoidis (*Zhi Zi*), and Herba Cephalanoploris (*Xiao Ji*). For the treatment of vacuity fire flaring upward tooth pain and oral sores, Radix Achyranthis Bidentatae can be combined with uncooked Radix Rehmanniae (*Sheng Di*), Tuber Ophiopogonis Japonici (*Mai Men Dong*), Rhizoma Anemarrhenae Aspheloidis (*Zhi Mu*), and Gypsum Fibrosum (*Shi Gao*) as in *Yu Nu Jian* (Jade Maiden Decoction). For the treatment of yin vacuity yang hyperactivity headache and dizziness, Radix Achyranthis Bidentatae can be combined with Haemititum (*Dai Zhe Shi*), uncooked Concha Ostreae (*Mu Li*), Radix Albus Paeoniae Lactiflorae (*Bai Shao*), and Radix Scrophulariae Ningpoensis (*Xuan Shen*) as in *Zhen Gan Xi Feng Tang* (Settle the Liver & Extinguish Wind Decoction).

Dosage: 6-15g. In larger doses, this ingredient can be used up to 30g.

Method of use: Decoct in water and administer internally. Radix Achyranthis Bidentatae (*Huai Niu Xi*) is better for supplementing and boosting the liver and kidneys, while Radix Cyathulae (*Chuan Niu Xi*) is stronger for quickening the blood and freeing the flow of the channels. Therefore, depending on the disease and following the symptoms, one should choose one or the other.

Cautions & contraindications: This medicinal is contraindicated in pregnant women and those with excessively profuse menstruation.

Squama Manitis Pentadactylis (*Chuan Shan Jia*)

Nature & flavor: Salty and slightly cold

Channel entry: Liver and stomach

Functions: Quickens the blood and frees the flow of the channels, descends the milk, disperses swelling and expels pus

Indications:

1. Used for blood stagnation blocked menstruation, concretions, conglomerations, accumulations, and lumps, and wind damp impediment pain. For the treatment of menstrual block, Squama Manitis Pentadactylis can be combined with Radix Angelicae Sinensis (*Dang Gui*), Radix Ligustici Wallichii (*Chuan Xiong*), Radix Achyranthis Bidentatae (*Niu Xi*), and Flos Carthami Tinctorii (*Hong Hua*). For the treatment of concretions and conglomerations, it can be combined with Rhizoma Sparganii (*San Leng*) and Rhizoma Curcumae Zedoariae (*E Zhu*). For the treatment of impediment pain, Squama Manitis Pentadactylis can be combined with Radix Et Rhizoma Notopterygii (*Qiang Huo*), Radix Ledebouriellae Divaricatae (*Fang Feng*), and Lignum Sappan (*Su Mu*).

2. Used for non-free flow of the breast milk, Squama Manitis Pentadactylis is commonly combined with Semen Vaccariae Segetalis (*Wang Bu Liu Xing*). If there is simultaneous liver depression breast distention, it may be combined with Radix Bupleuri (*Chai Hu*) and Pericarpium Citri Reticulatae Viride (*Qing Pi*). If lactation is scanty postpartum due to qi and blood insufficiency, it should be combined with Radix Astragali Membranacei (*Huang Qi*) and Radix Angelicae Sinensis (*Dang Gui*).

3. Used for sore and welling abscess swelling and pain. During the initial stage when there is no production of pus, Squama Manitis Pentadactylis is commonly combined with Flos Lonicerae Japonicae (*Jin Yin Hua*), Radix Trichosanthis Kirlowii (*Tian Hua Fen*), and Radix Rubrus Paeoniae Lactiflorae (*Chi Shao*) as in *Xian Fang Huo Ming Yin* (Immortal Formula Quicken the Destiny Drink). If pus has been produced but there is not rupture, Squama Manitis Pentadactylis is commonly combined with Spina Gleditschiae Chinensis (*Zao Jiao Ci*), Radix Angelicae Sinensis (*Dang Gui*), and Radix Astragali Membranacei (*Huang Qi*) as in *Tuo Nong San* (Out-thrust Pus Powder).

Dosage: 3-10g. One to1.5g each time when swallowed as a powder.

Method of use: Decoct in water and administer internally. Squama Manitis Pentadactylis can also be ground into powder and swallowed. Its therapeutic effect is better when ground into powder and swallowed.

Cautions & contraindications: This medicinal is contraindicated in pregnant women and for welling and flat abscess which have already ruptured.

Herba Lycopi Lucidi (*Ze Lan*)

Nature & flavor: Bitter, acrid, and slightly warm

Channel entry: Liver and spleen

Functions: Quickens the blood and transforms stasis, moves water and disperses swelling

Indications:

1. Used for menstrual irregularity, blocked menstruation, painful menstruation, and postpartum static blood abdominal pain, Herba Lycopi Lucidi is often combined with Radix Ligustici Wallichii (*Chuan Xiong*) and Radix Angelicae Sinensis (*Dang Gui*).

2. Used for water swelling. For water swelling with accompanying symptoms of heat, Herba Lycopi Lucidi can be combined with Rhizoma Imperatae Cylindricae (*Bai Mao Gen*). For postpartum water swelling, it may be combined with Radix Stephaniae Tetrandrae (*Han Fang Ji*).

Dosage: 6-12g

Method of use: Decoct in water and administer internally.

Rhizoma Curcumae Zedoariae (*E Zhu*)

Nature & flavor: Acrid, bitter, and warm

Channel entry: Liver and spleen

Functions: Moves the qi and breaks the blood, disperses accumulations and stops pain

Indications:

1. Used for concretions, conglomerations, glomus, and lumps and static blood blocked menstruation, Rhizoma Curcumae Zedoariae is commonly combined with Rhizoma Sparganii (*San Leng*).

2. Used for food accumulation distention and pain, Rhizoma Curcumae Zedoariae is commonly combined with Radix Auklandiae Lappae (*Mu Xiang*).

3. Used for menstrual irregularity and menstrual pain due to qi stagnation blood stasis, this medicinal can be combined with Radix Angelicae Sinensis (*Dang Gui*), Radix Rubrus Paeoniae Lactiflorae (*Chi Shao*), and Radix Ligustici Wallichii (*Chuan Xiong*).

Dosage: 4.5-10g

Method of use: Decoct in water and administer internally. Vinegar stir-frying is able to increase and strengthen this medicinal's effect of stopping pain and dispersing stasis.

Cautions & contraindications: This medicinal is contraindicated in pregnant women. Use cautiously in case of excessively profuse menstruation.

Rhizoma Sparganii (*San Leng*)

Nature & flavor: Acrid, bitter, and level

Channel entry: Liver and spleen

Functions: Breaks the blood and moves the qi, disperses accumulations and stops pain

Indications:

1. Used for concretions, conglomerations, glomus, and lumps and static blood blocked menstruation, Rhizoma Sparganii is commonly combined with Rhizoma Curcumae Zedoariae (*E Zhu*).

2. Used for food accumulation distention and pain, Rhizoma Sparganii is commonly combined with Radix Auklandiae Lappae (*Mu Xiang*), Semen Arecae Catechu (*Bing Lang*), Pericarpium Citri Reticulatae Viride (*Qing Pi*), and Massa Medica Fermentata (*Shen Qu*).

Dosage: 3-10g

Method of use: Decoct in water and administer internally.

Cautions & contraindications: This medicinal is contraindicated for use in pregnant women. Use cautiously in vacuity conditions so as to prevent damaging the righteous qi.

Resina Olibani (*Ru Xiang*)

Nature & flavor: Acrid, bitter, and warm

Channel entry: Heart, liver, and spleen

Functions: Quickens the blood and stops pain, disperses swelling and engenders muscle, *i.e.*, flesh, extends the sinews and quickens the network vessels

Indications:

1. Used for fall and strike swelling and pain due to blood stasis, Resina Olibani is commonly combined with Resina Myrrhae (*Mo Yao*) and Lignum Sappan (*Su Mu*).

2. Used for welling and flat abscess swelling and pain or enduring ulcers which will not close, it can be administered internally with Resina Myrrhae (*Mo Yao*), Realgar (*Xiong Huang*), and Secretio Moschi Moschiferi (*She Xiang*) and it can be applied externally with Resina Myrrhae (*Mo Yao*).

3. Used for wind damp impediment pain with sinew contracture, Resina Olibani is commonly combined with Radix Et Rhizoma Notopterygii (*Qiang Huo*) and Radix Angelicae Sinensis (*Dang Gui*).

Dosage: 3-10g. Externally, use a suitable amount.

Method of use: Decoct in water and administer internally or dissolve in alcohol to make into a tincture for external application. This medicinal may also be powdered and applied externally to sores whose mouths will not constrain, *i.e.*, close.

Cautions & contraindications: This medicinal is contraindicated for use in pregnant women.

Resina Myrrhae (*Mo Yao*)

Nature & flavor: Bitter and level

Channel entry: Liver channel

Functions: Scatters the blood and dispels stasis, disperses swelling and stabilizes pain

Indications:

1. Used for sinew and bone detriment and damage, Resina Myrrhae can be combined with Resina Olibani (*Ru Xiang*), powdered, mixed into a paste with alcohol, and applied to the affected area.

2. Used for unbearable heart and abdominal aching and pain, Resina Myrrhae can be combined with Resina Olibani (*Ru Xiang*), Squama Manitis Pentadactylis (*Chuan Shan Jia*), and Semen Momordicae Cochinensis (*Mu Bei Zi*).

Dosage: 3-12g. Externally, use a suitable amount.

Method of use: Decoct in water and administer or dissolve in alcohol to make into a tincture for external application. This medicinal may also be powdered and applied to sores whose mouth will not constrain, *i.e.*, close.

Semen Vaccariae Segetalis (*Wang Bu Liu Xing*)

Nature & flavor: Sweet, bitter, and level

Channel entry: Liver and stomach

Functions: Quickens the blood and frees the flow of the channels, descends the breast milk and disperses swelling

Indications:

1. Used for non-descension of the breast milk, Semen Vaccariae Segetalis can be combined with Medulla Tetrapanacis Papyriferi (*Tong Cao*), Radix Astragali Membranacei (*Huang Qi*), and Radix Angelicae Sinensis (*Dang Gui*) is due to qi and blood dual vacuity. If due to qi stagnation, Semen Vaccariae Segetalis can be combined with Squama Manitis Pentadactylis (*Chuan Shan Jia*). For the treatment of breast abscess, this medicinal can be combined with Herba Taraxaci Mongolici Cum Radice (*Pu Gong Ying*).

2. Used for blocked menstruation and painful menstruation, Semen Vaccariae Segetalis is commonly combined with Squama Manitis Pentadactylis (*Chuan Shan Jia*), Radix Angelicae Sinensis (*Dang Gui*), and Radix Ligustici Wallichii (*Chuan Xiong*).

In recent years, this medicinal has also been used for the treatment of post-herpetic neuralgia associated blood stasis when stir-fried, powdered, and mixed with sesame oil for external application to the affected area as long as there are no open sores.

Dosage: 4.5-10g. Externally, use a suitable amount.

Method of use: Decoct in water and administer internally or stir-fry, powder, mix with sesame oil, and apply externally.

Sanguis Draconis (*Xue Jie*)

Nature & flavor: Sweet, salty, and level

Channel entry: Heart and liver

Functions: Scatters stasis and stabilizes pain, stops bleeding and engenders muscle, *i.e.*, flesh

Indications:

1. Used for sinew and bone detriment and damage with unbearable aching and pain, Sanguis Draconis can be combined with Resina Myrrhae (*Mo Yao*), Radix Angelicae Sinensis (*Dang Gui*), Radix Angelicae Dahuricae (*Bai Zhi*), and Radix Rubrus Paeoniae Lactiflorae (*Chi Shao*).

2. Used for blood lumps within the abdomen, Sanguis Draconis can be combined with Resina Myrrhae (*Mo Yao*), Talcum (*Hua Shi*), and Cortex Radicis Moutan (*Dan Pi*).

3. Used for nasal spontaneous ejection of blood, Sanguis Draconis can be combined with Pollen Typhae (*Pu Huang*), ground into powder, and blown up the nostrils.

4. Used for scrofula which has already ruptured with unstoppable pus and water, Sanguis Draconis can be combined with carbonized Fructus Zizyphi Jujubae (*Da Zao*) and dry Radix Rehmanniae (*Gan Di Huang*), ground into powder, made into a paste, and applied externally to the affected area. This is called *Xue Jie San* (Dragon's Blood Powder).

Dosage: 0.5-1.5g each time when powdered and swallowed with other medicinals. Externally, use a suitable amount.

Method of use: Powder and wash down with water or other decocted medicinals. This medicinal may also be dissolved in alcohol to make into a tincture for external application.

Cautions & contraindications: This medicinal is contraindicated in pregnant women.

Lignum Sappan (*Su Mu*)

Nature & flavor: Sweet, salty, and level

Channel entry: Heart and liver

Functions: Moves the blood and dispels stasis, disperses swelling and stops pain

Indications:

1. Used for blocked menstruation, painful menstruation, and postpartum stasis obstruction, Lignum Sappan can be combined with Radix Angelicae Sinensis (*Dang Gui*) and Radix Ligustici Wallichii (*Chuan Xiong*).

2. Used for external injury due to fall and strike with swelling and pain, Lignum Sappan can be combined with Resina Olibani (*Ru Xiang*) and Resina Myrrhae (*Mo Yao*).

Dosage: 3-10g. Externally, use a suitable amount.

Method of use: Decoct in water and administer internally or dissolve in alcohol to make into a tincture for external application.

Cautions & contraindications: This medicinal is contraindicated for use in pregnant women.

Feces Trogopterori Seu Pteromi (*Wu Ling Zhi*)

Nature & flavor: Bitter, sweet, and warm

Channel entry: Liver and spleen

Functions: Moves the blood, stops pain, stops bleeding

Indications:

1. Used for menstrual irregularity and painful menstruation due to qi stagnation blood stasis and the discharge of dark clots, Feces Trogopterori Seu Pteromi is commonly combined with Pollen Typhae (*Pu Huang*) as in *Shi Xiao San* (Loose a Smile Powder).

2. Used for women's flooding and leaking and excessively profuse menstruation due to blood stasis, Feces Trogopterori Seu Pteromi can be combined with Gelatinum Corii Asini (*E Jiao*) and Radix Angelicae Sinensis (*Dang Gui*).

3. Used for stomach and abdominal piercing pain due to blood stasis and cold coagulation, Feces Trogopterori Seu Pteromi can be combined with blast-fried Rhizoma Zingiberis (*Pao Jiang*).

Dosage: 3-10g

Method of use: Decoct in water and administer internally. For quickening the blood use vinegar stir-fried. For stopping bleeding, use stir-fried till carbonized.

Cautions & contraindications: Use cautiously in pregnant women. This medicinal opposes or reverses Radix Panacis Ginseng (*Ren Shen*).

Eupolyphaga Seu Ophistoplatia (*Zhe Chong*)

Nature & flavor: Salty and cold. Has small toxins.

Channel entry: Liver, heart, and spleen

Functions: Breaks static blood, connects the sinews and bones

Indications:

1. Used for fall and strike pain, swelling, and fracture, Eupolyphaga Seu Ophistoplatia can be combined with Resina Olibani (*Ru Xiang*), Resina Myrrhae (*Mo Yao*), and Pyritum (*Zi Ran Tong*).

2. Used for blood stasis blocked menstruation and concretions, conglomerations, glomus, and lumps, Eupolyphaga Seu Ophistoplatia can be combined with Pollen Typhae (*Pu Huang*) and Feces Trogopterori Seu Pteromi (*Wu Ling Zhi*).

Dosage: 5-10g. Externally, use a suitable amount.

Method of use: Decoct in water and administer internally or soak in alcohol to make into a tincture for external application.

Cautions & contraindications: This medicinal is contraindicated in pregnant women.

Pyritum (*Zi Ran Tong*)

Nature & flavor: Acrid and level

Channel entry: Liver and kidneys

Functions: Scatters stasis, connects the bones, and stops pain

Indications: Used for fall and strike swelling and pain, breaks and injuries of the sinews and bones, Pyritum is often combined with Resina Olibani (*Ru Xiang*) and Resina Myrrhae (*Mo Yao*).

Dosage: 1-3g. Externally, use a suitable amount.

Method of use: This medicinal is mostly taken in pills and powders. It is not appropriate for decoction.

Spina Gleditschiae Chinensis (*Zao Jiao Ci*)

Nature & flavor: Acrid and warm

Channel entry: Liver and stomach

Functions: Disperses swelling and expels pus, treats wind and kills worms

Indications:
1. Used for welling and flat sores and swellings, breast abscesses, and scrofulous phlegm kernels, Spina Gleditschiae Chinensis is commonly combined with Squama Manitis Pentadactylis (*Chuan Shan Jia*), Flos Lonicerae Japonicae (*Jin Yin Hua*), and uncooked Radix Glycyrrhizae (*Gan Cao*).

2. Used for urticaria and skin itching, this ingredient can be boiled in oil and then the resulting oil applied externally.

In addition, in recent times, this medicinal is commonly used for the treatment of ovarian cysts and in order to promote ovulation.

Dosage: 3-10g. Externally, use a suitable amount.

Method of use: Decoct in water and administer internally.

12

Spirit-quieting medicinals

Medicinals whose main action is to quiet and stabilize the spirit will are called spirit-quieting medicinals. Spirit-quieting medicinals are divided into settling, stilling spirit-quieters and heart-nourishing spirit-quieters. They are mainly used for heart qi vacuity, heart blood vacuity, or heart fire hyperactivity and exuberance resulting in heart spirit restlessness, heart palpitations, racing heart, insomnia, profuse dreams, and even fright wind, epilepsy, and mania.

When heavy, settling, spirit-quieting medicinals made from mineral substances are used, these should be combined with stomach-nourishing, spleen-fortifying ingredients and they should not be administered for prolonged periods of time so as to prevent detriment damage of the stomach qi.

Cinnabar (*Zhu Sha*)

Nature & flavor: Sweet and cold. Has toxins.

Channel entry: Heart

Functions: Settles the heart and quiets the spirit, clears heat and resolves toxins

Indications:

1. Used for heart fire hyperactivity and exuberance resulting in heart spirit restlessness, vexatious heat within the chest, fright palpitations, racing heart, insomnia, and profuse dreams, Cinnabar is commonly combined with Rhizoma Coptidis Chinensis (*Huang Lian*) and uncooked Radix Rehmanniae (*Sheng Di*) as in *Zhu Sha An Shen Wan* (Cinnabar Quiet the Spirit Pills). For the treatment of blood vacuity heart palpitations and insomnia, Cinnabar should be combined with Radix Angelicae Sinensis (*Dang Gui*), Semen Zizyphi Spinosae (*Suan Zao Ren*), and Semen Biotae Orientalis (*Bai Zi Ren*). For the treatment of fright wind and epilepsy, Cinnabar can be combined with Succium (*Hu Po*) and Buthus Martensis (*Quan Xie*).

2. Used for sores and open sores swelling and toxins, Cinnabar is commonly combined with Realgar (*Xiong Huang*). These may be both administered internally and applied externally. For the treatment of throat swelling and pain or sores in the mouth and on the

tongue, Cinnabar can be combined with Borneolum (*Bing Pian*) and Borax (*Peng Sha*) and applied externally as in *Bing Peng San* (Borneol & Borax Powder).

Dosage: 0.3-1g. Externally, use a suitable amount.

Method of use: Cinnabar is taken in powders and pills. It may also be ground into powder and washed down. It can also be decocted and taken with other medicinals.

Cautions & contraindications: One should not take too large a dose of this medicinal internally nor should it be taken continuously for a long time. It should be used cautiously in those whose liver and kidney functions are abnormal.

Semen Zizyphi Spinosae (*Suan Zao Ren*)

Nature & flavor: Sweet and level

Channel entry: Heart and liver

Functions: Nourishes the heart and quiets the spirit, boosts yin and stops sweating

Indications:

1. Used for heart-liver blood vacuity leading to the arising of insomnia, profuse dreams, fright palpitations, and racing heart, Semen Zizyphi Spinosae can be combined with Radix Angelicae Sinensis (*Dang Gui*), Radix Albus Paeoniae Lactiflorae (*Bai Shao*), Radix Polygoni Multiflori (*He Shou Wu*), and Arillus Euphoriae Longanae (*Long Yan Rou*). For the treatment of liver vacuity with heat and vacuity vexation and insomnia, Semen Zizyphi Spinosae is commonly combined with Rhizoma Anemarrhenae Aspeloidis (*Zhi Mu*) and Sclerotium Poriae Cocos (*Fu Ling*) as in *Suan Zao Ren Tang* (Zizyphus Spinosa Decoction). For heart and kidneys not interacting or yin vacuity yang hyperactivity resulting in insomnia, heart palpitations, impaired memory, profuse dreams, and a dry mouth and throat, Semen Zizyphi Spinosae is commonly combined with uncooked Radix Rehmanniae (*Sheng Di*), Radix Scrophulariae Ningpoensis (*Xuan Shen*), and Semen Biotae Orientalis (*Bia Zi Ren*) as in *Tian Wang Bu Xin Dan* (Heavenly Emperor Supplement the Heart Elixir).

2. Used for bodily vacuity spontaneous perspiration and night sweats, Semen Zizyphi Spinosae is commonly combined with Radix Codonopsitis Pilosulae (*Dang Shen*), Fructus Schisandrae Chinensis (*Wu Wei Zi*), and Fructus Corni Officinalis (*Shan Zhu Yu*).

Dosage: 10-18g. One-and-a-half to 3g each time when swallowed as a powder.

Method of use: Decoct in water and administer internally. It may also be ground into powder and swallowed before sleep.

Semen Biotae Orientalis (*Bai Zi Ren*)

Nature & flavor: Sweet and level

Channel entry: Heart, kidneys, and large intestine

Functions: Nourishes the heart and quiets the spirit, moistens the intestines and frees the flow of the stool

Indications:

1. Used for blood not nourishing the heart leading to the arising of vacuity vexation insomnia, fright palpitations, and racing heart, Semen Biotae Orientalis is commonly combined with Semen Zizyphi Spinosae (*Suan Zao Ren*), Fructus Schisandrae Chinensis (*Wu Wei Zi*), and Sclerotium Poriae Cocos (*Fu Ling*) as in *Yang Xin Tang* (Nourish the Heart Decoction).

2. Used for yin vacuity blood scantiness intestinal dryness constipation, Semen Biotae Orientalis is commonly combined with Semen Pruni (*Yu Li Ren*) and Semen Pruni Persicae (*Tao Ren*) as in *Wu Ren Wan* (Five Seeds Pills).

Dosage: 10-18g

Method of use: Decoct in water and administer internally.

Cautions & contraindications: Use cautiously in case of loose stools or profuse phlegm.

Radix Polygalae Tenuifoliae (*Yuan Zhi*)

Nature & flavor: Acrid, bitter, and slightly warm

Channel entry: Lungs and heart

Functions: Calms the heart and quiets the spirit, dispels phlegm and opens the orifices, disperses welling abscesses and scatters nodulations

Indications:

1. Used for heart spirit restlessness, fright palpitations, insomnia, and impaired memory. For the treatment of fright palpitations, Radix Polygalae Tenuifoliae can be combined with Cinnabar (*Zhu Sha*) and Dens Draconis (*Long Chi*) as in *Yuan Zhi Wan* (Polygala Pills). For the treatment of insomnia and impaired memory, Radix Polygalae Tenuifoliae can be combined with Radix Panacis Ginseng (*Ren Shen*) and Rhizoma Acori Graminei (*Shi Chang Pu*) as in *Bu Wang San* (No Memory Powder).

2. Used for phlegm obstructing the heart portals resulting in essence spirit confusion and chaos, spirit will abstraction, and fright epilepsy, Radix Polygalae Tenuifoliae is commonly combined with Rhizoma Acori Graminei (*Shi Chang Pu*), Tuber Curcumae (*Yu Jin*), and Alum (*Bai Fan*).

3. Used for cough with profuse phlegm which is thick and difficult to spit out, Radix Polygalae Tenuifoliae can be combined with Semen Pruni Armeniacae (*Xing Ren*), Radix Platycodi Grandiflori (*Jie Geng*), and Radix Glycyrrhizae (*Gan Cao*).

4. Used for welling and flat abcesses swelling and toxins and breast swelling and pain, Radix Polygalae Tenuifoliae can be used alone as a powder or taken with yellow, *i.e.*, rice wine. This mixture may also be applied externally.

Dosage: 3-10g. Externally, use a suitable amount.

Method of use: Decoct in water and administer internally.

Cautions & contraindications: Use cautiously in those with ulcer disease and gastritis.

Cortex Albizziae Julibrissinis (*He Huan Pi*)

Nature & flavor: Sweet and level

Channel entry: Heart and liver

Functions: Resolves depression and quiets the mind, quickens the blood and disperses swelling

Indications:

1. Used for insomnia, profuse dreams, easy anger, chest oppression, scanty eating, and emotional depression due to liver depression qi stagnation, Cortex Albizziae Julibrissinis

can be combined with Radix Salviae Miltiorrhizae (*Dan Shen*) and Caulis Polygoni Multiflori (*Ye Jiao Teng*).

2. Used for fall and strike injury and pain, Cortex Albizziae Julibrissinis can be combined with Resina Olibani (*Ru Xiang*) and Resina Myrrhae (*Mo Yao*).

3. Used for lung abscess, Cortex Albizziae Julibrissinis can be combined with Semen Benincasae Hispidae (*Dong Gua Ren*), Herba Houttuyniae Cordatae Cum Radice (*Yu Xing Cao*), and Semen Pruni Persicae (*Tao Ren*).

4. Used for the pain of unruptured sores and swellings, this medicinal can be combined with Herba Taraxaci Mongolici Cum Radice (*Pu Gong Ying*), Spina Gleditschiae Chinensis (*Zao Jiao Ci*), and Squama Manitis Pentadactylis (*Chuan Shan Jia*).

Dosage: 10-15g

Method of use: Decoct in water and administer internally.

Caulis Polygoni Multiflori (*Ye Jiao Teng*)

Nature & flavor: Sweet and level

Channel entry: Heart and liver

Functions: Nourishes the blood and quiets the spirit, dispels wind and frees the flow of the network vessels

Indications:

1. Used for heart blood vacuity insomnia, fright palpitations, and profuse dreams, Caulis Polygoni Multiflori is commonly combined with Semen Zizyphi Spinosae (*Suan Zao Ren*) and Semen Biotae Orientalis (*Bai Zi Ren*).

2. Used for blood vacuity generalized body pain and wind damp impediment pain, Caulis Polygoni Multiflori can be combined with Radix Angelicae Sinensis (*Dang Gui*), Caulis Milletiae Seu Spatholobi (*Ji Xue Teng*), and Radix Salviae Miltiorrhizae (*Dan Shen*).

In addition, this medicinal can be used as an external wash for the treatment of itching.

Dosage: 10-15g. Externally, use a suitable amount.

Method of use: Decoct in water and administer internally or use as a wash externally.

13

Liver-leveling, wind-extinguishing medicinals

Medicinals whose main action is to level and extinguish liver wind or level the liver and subdue yang are called liver-leveling medicinals. The effect of these medicinals is to level the liver and subdue yang, extinguish wind and stop tetany. They are mainly appropriate for use in ascendant liver yang hyperactivity dizziness and vertigo and liver wind stirring internally tetany, spasms and contractures, and convulsions. Some of the medicinals in this class also have the effect of clearing the liver and are appropriate for use in liver heat red, swollen, painful eyes and headache.

Some of the medicinals in this category are cold and some are warm and thus their use should be differentiated. Medicinals which are cold or cool in nature are not appropriate for use in spleen vacuity chronic fright convulsions, while medicinals which are warm and dry in nature should be used cautiously in case of yin vacuity yang hyperactivity.

Cornu Antelopis Saiga-tatarici (*Ling Yang Jiao*)[7]

Nature & flavor: Salty and cold

Channel entry: Liver and heart

Functions: Levels the liver and extinguishes wind, clears the liver and brightens the eyes, clears heat and resolves toxins

Indications:

1. Used for liver wind stirring internally with fright epilepsy and convulsions, especially when extreme heat is stirring the wind, Cornu Antelopis Saiga-tatarici can be combined with Ramulus Uncariae Cum Uncis (*Gou Teng*), Flos Chrysanthemi Morifolii (*Ju Hua*), and uncooked Radix Rehmanniae (*Sheng Di*) as in *Ling Jiao Gou Teng Tang* (Antelope & Uncaria Decoction).

---

[7] Saiga antelope is an endangered species and its horn should not be used for the manufacture of medicine. It can be substituted by Cornu Caprae (*Shan Yang Jiao*) or goat horn.

2. Used for ascendant liver yang hyperactivity resulting in dizziness and vertigo, Cornu Antelopis Saiga-tatarici can be combined with Flos Chrysanthemi Morifolii (*Ju Hua*) and Concha Haliotidis (*Shi Jue Ming*).

3. Used for liver fire flaring upward resulting in headache and red eyes, Cornu Antelopis Saiga-tatarici is commonly combined with Semen Cassiae Torae (*Jue Ming Zi*), Radix Scutellariae Baicalensis (*Huang Qin*), and Radix Gentianae Scabrae (*Long Dan Cao*) as in *Ling Yang Jiao San* (Antelope Horn Powder).

4. Used for warm heat disease with strong fever and spirit clouding, delirious speech, agitation, and mania or for heat toxin emission of macules, Cornu Antelopis Saiga-tatarici can be combined with Cornu Rhinocerotis (*Xi Jiao*) and Gypsum Fibrosum (*Shi Gao*) as in *Zi Xue San* (Purple Snow Powder).

Dosage: 3-6g. When taken as a powder, take 0.6-1.5g each time.

Method administration: Decoct alone first, then add to other decocted medicinals and administer. It can also be ground in water to obtain and liquid or taken internally as powder.

Calculus Bovis (*Niu Huang*)

Nature & flavor: Bitter and cool

Channel entry: Liver and heart

Functions: Extinguishes wind and stops tetany, transforms phlegm and opens the orifices, clears heat and resolves toxins

Indications:

1. Used for warm heat disease with high fever, spirit clouding, tetany, tremors, and convulsions, and acute pediatric fright wind, Calculus Bovis is commonly combined with Cinnabar (*Zhu Sha*), Buthus Martensis (*Quan Xie*), and Ramulus Uncariae Cum Uncis (*Gou Teng*) as in *Niu Huang San* (Cow Bezoar Powder).

2. Used for warm heat disease heat entering the pericardium resulting in spirit clouding, delirious speech and even wind stroke, fright wind, and epilepsy categorized as phlegm heat internal blockage, Calculus Bovis is commonly combined with Secretio Moschi Moschiferi (*She Xiang*), Borneolum (*Bing Pian*), Fructus Gardeniae Jasminoidis (*Zhi Zi*), and Rhizoma Coptidis Chinensis (*Huang Lian*) as in *An Gong Niu Huang Wan* (Quiet the Palace Cow Bezoar Pills).

3. Used for heat toxins brewing and binding resulting in throat swelling and pain, ulceration, sores in the mouth and on the tongue, welling and flat abscesses, and clove sore toxins, Calculus Bovis is commonly combined with Radix Scutellariae Baicalensis (*Huang Qin*) and Realgar (*Xiong Huang*) as in *Niu Huang Jie Du Wan* (Cow Bezoar Resolve Toxins Pills). For the treatment of breast rock and scrofula, it can be combined with Secretio Moschi Moschiferi (*She Xiang*), Resina Olibani (*Ru Xiang*) and Resina Myrrhae (*Mo Yao*) as in *Xi Huang Wan* (Rhinoceros Horn & Cow Bezoar Pills).

Dosage: 0.2-0.5g. Externally, use a suitable amount.

Method of use: Taken in pills and powders. It is not appropriate to decoct this medicinal.

Cautions & contraindications: Use cautiously in pregnant women. It is not appropriate to use this medicinal in those with replete heat patterns.

Os Draconis (*Long Gu*)

Nature & flavor: Sweet, astringent, and slightly cold

Channel entry: Heart and liver

Functions: Levels the liver and subdues yang, settles, stills, and quiets the spirit, restrains, constrains, secures, and astringes, engenders muscles and constrains sores

Indications:

1. Used for yin vacuity yang hyperactivity resulting in vexation and agitation, easy anger, and dizziness and vertigo, Os Draconis can be combined with Concha Ostreae (*Mu Li*), Radix Albus Paeoniae Lactiflorae (*Chi Shao*), and Haemititum (*Dai Zhe Shi*) as in *Zhen Gan Xi Feng Tang* (Settle the Liver & Extinguish Wind Decoction).

2. Used for spirit will restlessness, heart palpitations, and insomnia as well as fright epilepsy and mania and withdrawal. If agitation and stirring are due to yang qi, Os Draconis can be combined with Cinnabar (*Zhu Sha*) and Magnetitum (*Ci Shi*). If due to yin and blood insufficiency, it may be combined with Semen Zizyphi Spinosae (*Suan Zao Ren*), cooked Radix Rehmanniae (*Shu Di*), and Radix Angelicae Sinensis (*Dang Gui*). If due to heart qi insufficiency, it may be combined with Radix Panacis Ginseng (*Ren Shen*), Sclerotium Poriae Cocos (*Fu Ling*), and Radix Polygalae Tenuifoliae (*Yuan Zhi*).

3. Used for seminal emission, abnormal vaginal discharge, vacuity sweating, and flooding and leaking. For the treatment of kidney vacuity seminal emission, Os Draconis can be combined with Concha Ostreae (*Mu Li*), Semen Astragali Complanati (*Sha Yuan Zi*), and Semen Euryalis Ferocis (*Qian Shi*) as in *Jin Suo Gu Jing Wan* (Golden Lock Secure the Essence Pills). For the treatment of flooding and leaking and abnormal vaginal discharge, Os Draconis can be combined with Concha Ostreae (*Mu Li*), Os Sepiae Seu Sepiellae (*Wu Zei Gu*), and Radix Dioscoreae Oppositae (*Shan Yao*). For vacuity sweating, it is commonly combined with Concha Ostreae (*Mu Li*) and Fructus Schisandrae Chinensis (*Wu Wei Zi*).

4. Used for sores and open sores which do not heal for a long time after rupturing, damp sore itching, and metal sore bleeding , *i.e.*, bleeding due to cuts, Os Draconis can be powdered, combined with Alum (*Ku Fan*), and applied externally to the affected area.

Dosage: 10-30g. Externally, use a suitable amount.

Method of use: When taken in decoction, this medicinal should be decocted first. For leveling the liver and subduing yang, settling, stilling, and quieting the spirit, use uncooked. For restraining, constraining, securing, and astringing, engendering muscle and constraining sores, one should use calcined.

Concha Ostreae (*Mu Li*)

Nature & flavor: Salty, astringent, and slightly cold

Channel entry: Liver and kidneys

Functions: Levels the liver and subdues yang, softens the hard and scatters nodulations, restrains, constrains, secures, and astringes

Indications:

1. Used for yin vacuity yang hyperactivity resulting in vexation and agitation, restlessness, heart palpitations, insomnia, and dizziness and vertigo, Concha Ostreae is commonly combined with Os Draconis (*Long Gu*), Radix Achyranthis Bidentatae (*Niu Xi*), Radix Albus Paeoniae Lactiflorae (*Bai Shao*),and Haemititum (*Dai Zhe Shi*) as in *Zhen Gan Xi Feng Tang* (Settle the Liver & Extinguish Wind Decoction). For heat disease damaging yin resulting in vacuity wind stirring internally and tremors and convulsions of the hands and feet, Concha Ostreae is commonly combined with Plastrum Testudinis (*Gui Ban*), Carapax Amydae Sinensis (*Bie Jia*), uncooked Radix Rehmanniae (*Sheng Di*), and Gelatinum Corii Asini (*E Jiao*) as in *San Jia Fu Mai Tang* (Three Shells Restore the Pulse Decoction).

2. Used for phlegm fire depression and binding resulting in scrofula and phlegm kernels, Concha Ostreae is commonly combined with Bulbus Fritillariae Thunbergii (*Zhe Bei Mu*) and Radix Scrophulariae Ningpoensis (*Xuan Shen*) as in *Xiao Luo Wan* (Disperse Scrofula Pills). It can also be used for the treatment of hypochondral concretions and lumps. In this case, Concha Ostreae is commonly combined with Radix Salviae Miltiorrhizae (*Dan Shen*), Carapax Amydae Sinensis (*Bie Jia*), and Herba Lycopi Lucidi (*Ze Lan*).

3. Used for vacuity sweating, seminal emission, abnormal vaginal discharge, and flooding and leaking. For the treatment of spontaneous perspiration and night sweats, Concha Ostreae is commonly combined with Radix Astragali Membranacei (*Huang Qi*), Fructus Levis Tritici Aestivi (*Fu Xiao Mai*), and Radix Ephedrae (*Ma Huang Gen*) as in *Mu Li San* (Oyster Shell Powder). For the treatment of kidney vacuity seminal emission, Concha Ostreae is commonly combined with Semen Astragali Complanati (*Sha Yuan Zi*), Semen Euryalis Ferocis (*Qian Shi*), and Stamen Nelumbinis Nuciferae (*Lian Xu*) as in *Jin Suo Gu Jing Wan* (Golden Lock Secure the Essence Pills). For the treatment of abnormal vaginal discharge and flooding and leaking, it can be combined with Os Draconis (*Long Gu*), Os Sepiae Seu Sepiellae (*Wu Zei Gu*), and Radix Dioscoreae Oppositae (*Shan Yao*).

In addition, because this medicinal has an effect of controlling acidity, it can be used for excess stomach acid.

Dosage: 15-30g

Method of use: Crush and decoct first. For leveling the liver and subduing yang, softening the hard and scattering nodulations, one should use uncooked. For restraining, constraining, securing, and astringing and for controlling acidity, one should use calcined.

Haemititum (*Dai Zhe Shi*)

Nature & flavor: Bitter, sweet, and cold

Channel entry: Liver and heart

Functions: Levels the liver and subdues yang, settles counterflow and downbears the qi, cools the blood and stops bleeding

Indications:

1. Used for ascendant liver yang hyperactivity headache and dizziness, Haemititum is commonly combined with Os Draconis (*Long Gu*), Concha Ostreae (*Mu Li*), and Radix Albus Paeoniae Lactiflorae (*Bai Shao*) as in *Zhen Gan Xi Feng Tang* (Settle the Liver & Extinguish Wind Decoction).

179

2. Used for burping, hiccup, vomiting, and qi panting. For the treatment of stomach vacuity phlegm obstruction resulting in burping and vomiting, Haemititum is commonly combined with Flos Inulae Racemosae (*Xuan Fu Hua*), Rhizoma Pinelliae Ternatae (*Ban Xia*), uncooked Rhizoma Zingiberis (*Sheng Jiang*), and Radix Panacis Ginseng (*Ren Shen*) as in *Xuan Fu Dai Zhe Tang* (Inula & Hematite Decoction). For the treatment of lung-kidney dual vacuity resulting in qi counterflow panting respiration, Haemititum can be combined with Radix Codonopsitis Pilosulae (*Dang Shen*) and Fructus Corni Officinalis (*Shan Zhu Yu*) as in *Shen Zhe Zhen Qi Tang* (Ginseng & Hematite Settle the Qi Decoction).

3. Used for blood heat frenetic movement resulting in spitting of blood and spontaneous ejection of blood, Haemititum can be combined with Radix Albus Paeoniae Lactiflorae (*Bai Shao*), Caulis Bambusae In Taeniis (*Zhu Ru*), and Fructus Arctii Lappae (*Niu Bang Zi*) as in *Han Jiang Tang* (Cold Downbearing Decoction).

Dosage: 10-30g

Method administration: When taken in decoct, this medicinal should be decocted first. For downbearing counterflow and leveling the liver, it is ok to use uncooked. For stopping bleeding, it should be used calcined.

Cautions & contraindications: Use cautiously in pregnant women.

Concha Haliotidis (*Shi Jue Ming*)

Nature & flavor: Salty and cold

Channel entry: Liver and kidneys

Functions: Levels the liver and subdues yang, clears the liver and brightens the eyes

Indications:

1. Used for headache, dizziness, and red eyes due to ascendant liver yang hyperactivity and liver fire, Concha Haliotidis is commonly combined with Radix Achyranthis Bidentatae (*Niu Xi*), Rhizoma Gastrodiae Elatae (*Tian Ma*), and Ramulus Uncariae Cum Uncis (*Gou Teng*) as in *Tian Ma Gou Teng Yin* (Gastrodia & Uncariae Drink).

2. Used for eye screen and obstruction of vision, blurred vision, clear-eyed blindness, and sparrow eyes, *i.e.*, night blindness, Concha Haliotidis is commonly combined with cooked Radix Rehmanniae (*Shu Di*), Fructus Corni Officinalis (*Shan Zhu Yu*), and Fructus Lycii Chinensis (*Gou Qi Zi*) as in *Ming Mu Di Huang Wan* (Brighten the Eyes Rehmannia Pills).

Dosage: 10-30g

Method of use: Decoct in water and administer internally, adding first or take in powders and pills.

Cautions & contraindications: Use cautiously in case of spleen-stomach vacuity cold, poor digestion, and stomach acid deficiency.

Ramulus Uncariae Cum Uncis (*Gou Teng*)

Nature & flavor: Sweet and slightly cold

Channel entry: Liver and pericardium

Functions: Extinguishes wind and stops tetany, clears heat and levels the liver

Indications:

1. Used for fright epilepsy, tremors, and convulsions, Ramulus Uncariae Cum Uncis is often combined with Rhizoma Gastrodiae Elatae (*Tian Ma*), Buthus Martensis (*Quan Xie*), and Cornu Antelopis Saiga-tatarici (*Ling Yang Jiao*). If categorized as heat exuberance stirring of wind, Ramulus Uncariae Cum Uncis can be combined with Cornu Antelopis Saiga-tatarici (*Ling Yang Jiao*), Radix Gentianae Scabrae (*Long Dan Cao*), and Flos Chrysanthemi Morifolii (*Ju Hua*).

2. Used for liver fire flaring upward resulting in head distention, headache, and red, swollen, painful eyes, Ramulus Uncariae Cum Uncis is commonly combined with Spica Prunellae Vulgaris (*Xia Ku Cao*), Fructus Gardeniae Jasminoidis (*Zhi Zi*), and Radix Scutellariae Baicalensis (*Huang Qin*).

3. Used for ascendant liver yang hyperactivity dizziness and vertigo, Ramulus Uncariae Cum Uncis is commonly combined with Flos Chrysanthemi Morifolii (*Ju Hua*), Concha Haliotidis (*Shi Jue Ming*), and Radix Albus Paeoniae Lactiflorae (*Bai Shao*).

Dosage: 10-15g

Method of use: Decoct in water and administer internally. When taken in decoction, this medicinal should be added later and cooked for no more than 20 minutes. Otherwise, its downbearing of pressure action will be weakened and decreased.

Rhizoma Gastrodiae Elatae (*Tian Ma*)

Nature & flavor: Sweet and level

Channel entry: Liver

Functions: Extinguishes wind and stops tetany, levels the liver and subdues yang, frees the flow of the network vessels and stops pain

Indications:

1. Used for liver wind stirring internally fright epilepsy, tremors, and convulsions. For the treatment of pediatric high fever fright wind, Rhizoma Gastrodiae Elatae can be combined with Ramulus Uncariae Cum Uncis (*Gou Teng*), Cornu Antelopis Saiga-tatarici (*Ling Yang Jiao*), and Buthus Martensis (*Quan Xie*) as in *Gou Teng Yin* (Uncaria Drink). For the treatment of pediatric spleen vacuity chronic fright, it can be combined with Radix Panacis Ginseng (*Ren Shen*), Rhizoma Atractylodis Macrocephalae (*Bai Zhu*), and Bombyx Batryticatus (*Jiang Can*) as in *Xing Pi San* (Arouse the Spleen Powder). For the treatment of tetanus, Rhizoma Gastrodiae Elatae can be combined with Rhizoma Arisaematis (*Tian Nan Xing*), Radix Ledebouriellae Divaricatae (*Fang Feng*), and Radix Aconiti Coreani Seu Typhonii (*Bai Fu Zi*) as in *Yu Zhen San* (Jade True Powder).

2. Used for headache, dizziness, and vertigo. If due to ascendant liver yang hyperactivity, Rhizoma Gastrodiae Elatae can be combined with Ramulus Uncariae Cum Uncis (*Gou Teng*), Radix Scutellariae Baicalensis (*Huang Qin*), and Radix Achyranthis Bidentatae (*Niu Xi*) as in *Tian Ma Gou Teng Yin* (Gastrodia & Uncaria Drink). If due to wind phlegm harassing above, Rhizoma Gastrodiae Elatae can be combined with Rhizoma Pinelliae Ternatae (*Ban Xia*), Rhizoma Atractylodis Macrocephalae (*Bai Zhu*), and Sclerotium Poriae Cocos (*Fu Ling*) as in *Ban Xia Bai Zhu Tian Ma Tang* (Pinellia, Atractylodes & Gastrodia Decoction). If categorized as yin and blood insufficiency, Rhizoma Gastrodiae Elatae can be combined with Radix Angelicae Sinensis (*Dang Gui*), Radix Albus Paeoniae Lactiflorae (*Bai Shao*), and cooked Radix Rehmanniae (*Shu Di*). For the treatment of one-sided headache which sometimes occurs and sometimes stops and endures for days without healing, Rhizoma Gastrodiae Elatae is commonly combined with Radix Ligustici Wallichii (*Chuan Xiong*) as in *Tian Ma Wan* (Gastrodia Pills).

3. Used for wind damp impediment pain, numbness of the extremities, and non-use of the hands and feet, *i.e.*, paralysis, Rhizoma Gastrodiae Elatae is commonly combined with Radix Gentianae Macrophyllae (*Qin Jiao*), Radix Angelicae Pubescentis (*Du Huo*), Radix Achyranthis Bidentatae (*Niu Xi*), and Ramulus Loranthi Seu Visci (*Sang Ji Sheng*).

Dosage: 3-10g. When ground into powder and swallowed, 1-1.5g each time.

Method of use: Decoct in water and administer internally. It may also be ground into powder and swallowed.

Buthus Martensis (*Quan Xie*)

Nature & flavor: Sweet, acrid, and level. Has toxins.

Channel entry: Liver

Functions: Extinguishes wind and stops tetany, resolves toxins and scatters nodulations, frees the flow of the network vessels and stops pain

Indications:

1. Used for many types of causes resulting in tetany, tremors, and convulsions. For the treatment of acute pediatric fright wind, Buthus Martensis can be combined with Rhizoma Gastrodiae Elatae (*Tian Ma*), Ramulus Uncariae Cum Uncis (*Gou Teng*), and Cornu Antelopis Saiga-tatarici (*Ling Yang Jiao*). For the treatment of spleen vacuity chronic fright, it can be combined with Radix Codonopsitis Pilosulae (*Dang Shen*), Rhizoma Atractylodis Macrocephalae (*Bai Zhu*), and Rhizoma Gastrodiae Elatae (*Tian Ma*). For wind stroke with deviated eyes and mouth, Buthus Martensis is commonly combined with Radix Aconiti Coreani Seu Typhonii (*Bai Fu Zi*) and Bombyx Batryticatus (*Jiang Can*) as in *Qian Zheng San* (Pull Upright Powder). For the treatment of tetanus, it is often combined with Rhizoma Arisaematis (*Tian Nan Xing*) and Scolopendra Subspinipes (*Wu Gong*) as in *Wu Hu Zhui Feng San* (Five Tigers Expel Wind Powder).

2. Used for sores and open sores swelling and toxins and scrofulous binding and kernels, Buthus Martensis can be used alone, in which case it is roasted till scorched, ground into powder, and taken with yellow wine. Or it may be combined with Fructus Gardeniae Jasminoidis (*Zhi Zi*) fried till black in sesame oil. Then the dregs are removed, yellow wax is added ,and it is made into an ointment applied externally to the affected area.

3. Used for recalcitrant one-sided headache and wind damp impediment pain, Buthus Martensis can be used alone, ground into powder, and swallowed or combined with Scolopendra Subspinipes (*Wu Gong*) and Bombyx Batryticatus (*Jiang Can*).

Dosage: When swallowed after being ground into powder or in pills and powders, 0.5-1g each time. When decocted, one can administer up to 2-5g. Externally, use a suitable amount.

Cautions & contraindications: This ingredient has toxins. Therefore, the amount used should not be too large. Use cautiously in pregnant women and those with blood vacuity engendering wind.

Lumbricus (*Di Long*)

Nature & flavor: Salty and cold

Channel entry: Liver, kidneys, lungs, and urinary bladder

Functions: Clears heat and extinguishes wind, clears the lungs and levels panting, soothes the sinews and frees the flow of the network vessels, disinhibits urination and frees the flow of strangury

Indications:

1. Used for high fever vexation and agitation, fright wind tremors and convulsions, Lumbricus can be used alone or combined with Ramulus Uncariae Cum Uncis (*Gou Teng*), Bombyx Batryticatus (*Jiang Can*), and Cornu Antelopis Saiga-Tatarici (*Ling Yang Jiao*). For the treatment of phlegm fire harassing above mania, agitation, and restlessness, fresh Lumbricus can be used after being washed, dissolved in sugar water, and taken.

2. Used for lung heat blockage and exuberance resulting in panting respiration with phlegm sounds and yellow, sticky, thick phlegm, Lumbricus can be used alone after being powdered and taken or it may be combined with Herba Ephedrae (*Ma Huang*), Gypsum Fibrosum (*Shi Gao*), Semen Pruni Armeniacae (*Xing Ren*), and Radix Scutellariae Baicalensis (*Huang Qin*).

3. Used for heat impediment joint redness, swelling, heat, and pain with inhibited bending and extending, Lumbricus is commonly combined with Ramulus Mori Albi (*Sang Zhi*), Caulis Lonicerae Japonicae (*Ren Dong Teng*), Caulis Trachelospermi Jasminoidis (*Luo Shi Teng*), and Radix Rubrus Paeoniae Lactiflorae (*Chi Shao*). For cold damp impediment pain with inhibited bending and extending, Lumbricus should be combined with Radix Aconiti (*Chuan Wu*), Radix Aconiti (*Cao Wu*), Resina Olibani (*Ru Xiang*), and Resina Myrrhae (*Mo Yao*) as in *Xiao Huo Luo Dan* (Minor Quicken the Network Vessels Elixir). Lumbricus can also be used for qi vacuity blood stagnation with inhibition of the network vessels resulting in hemiplegia. In that case, it is commonly combined with Radix Astragali Membranacei (*Huang Qi*), Radix Angelicae Sinensis (*Dang Gui*), and Flos Carthami Tinctorii (*Hong Hua*) as in *Bu Yang Huan Wu Tang* (Supplement Yang Restore the Five [Viscera] Decoction).

4. Used for heat binding urinary block or urinary strangury, dribbling, astringency, and pain, Lumbricus can be used alone or combined with Semen Plantaginis (*Che Qian Zi*) and Caulis Akebiae (*Mu Tong*).

In addition, fresh Lumbricus can be mashed with sugar and applied externally for the treatment of acute parotitis, chronic lower limb ulcers, and injuries due to burns and scalds.

Dosage: 6-15g. When used fresh, one can use up to 10-20g. When ground into powder and swallowed, use 1-3g each time. Externally, use a suitable amount.

Method of use: Decoct in water and administer internally.

Bombyx Batryticatus (*Jiang Can*)

Nature & flavor: Salty, acrid, and level

Channel entry: Liver, lungs, and stomach

Functions: Dispels wind and stabilizes spasms, transforms phlegm and scatters nodulations

Indications:

1. Used for various types of spasms and contractures. For those due to phlegm heat, Bombyx Batryticatus can be combined with Calculus Bovis (*Niu Huang*), Rhizoma Coptidis Chinensis (*Huang Lian*), and bile-processed Rhizoma Arisaematis (*Dan Nan Xing*). For enduring convulsions in children due to spleen vacuity, Bombyx Batryticatus can be combined with Radix Codonopsitis Pilosulae (*Dang Shen*), Rhizoma Atractylodis Macrocephalae (*Bai Zhu*), and Rhizoma Gastrodiae Elatae (*Tian Ma*). For epilepsy, Bombyx Batryticatus can be combined with Buthus Martensis (*Quan Xie*), Sclopendra Suspinipes (*Wu Gong*), and Periostracum Cicadae (*Chan Tui*).

2. Used for throat swelling and pain, Bombyx Batryticatus can be combined with Radix Platycodi Grandiflori (*Jie Geng*), Herba Menthae Haplocalycis (*Bo He*), and Radix Glycyrrhizae (*Gan Cao*).

3. Used for scrofulous phlegm kernels, Bombyx Batryticatus can be combined with Spica Prunellae Vulgaris (*Xia Ku Cao*), Bulbus Fritillariae Thunbergii (*Zhe Bei Mu*), and Concha Ostreae (*Mu Li*).

4. Used for skin itching and wind rash, Bombyx Batryticatus is commonly combined with Periostracum Cicadae (*Chan Tui*) and Radix Ledebouriellae Divaricatae (*Fang Feng*).

Dosage: 3-10g

Method of use: Decoct in water and administer internally. Use stir-fried for better effect for transforming phlegm. For scattering wind heat, use uncooked.

Fructus Tribuli Terrestris (*Bai Ji Li*)

Nature & flavor: Acrid, bitter, and warm

Channel entry: Liver and lungs

Functions: Dispels wind and courses the liver, moves the qi and quickens the blood

Indications:

1. Used for ascendant liver yang hyperactivity headache, dizziness, and vertigo, Fructus Tribuli Terrestris is commonly combined with Ramulus Uncariae Cum Uncis (*Gou Teng*) and Radix Achyranthis Bidentatae (*Niu Xi*).

2. Used for breast distention and pain with itchy nipples, Fructus Tribuli Terrestris can be combined with Pericarpium Citri Reticulatae Viride (*Qing Pi*) and Rhizoma Cyperi Rotundi (*Xiang Fu*).

3. Used for wind heat resulting in itchy skin, Fructus Tribuli Terrestris can be combined with Periostracum Cicadae (*Chan Tui*) and Radix Ledebouriellae Divaricatae (*Fang Feng*).

4. Used for red, swollen , itchy eyes with excessive tearing due to liver heat and wind, Fructus Tribuli Terrestris can be combined with Semen Cassiae Torae (*Jue Ming Zi*) and Flos Chrysanthemi Morifolii (*Ju Hua*).

Dosage: 6-15g

Method of use: Decoct in water and administer internally.

Scolopendra Subspinipes (*Wu Gong*)

Nature & flavor: Acrid and warm. Has toxins.

Channel entry: Liver

Functions: Extinguishes wind and settles tetany, attacks toxins and scatters nodulations, frees the flow of the network vessels and stops pain

Indications:

1. Used for children's fright wind, spasms and contractures, tetany, wind stroke hemiplegia, and tetanus, Scolopendra Subspinipes is commonly combined with Buthus Martensis (*Quan Xie*), Bombyx Batryticatus (*Jiang Can*), and Ramulus Uncariae Cum Uncis (*Gou Teng*).

2. Used for sores and open sores, scrofula, and insect and snake bite injuries, Scolopendra Subspinipes can be combined with Radix Glycyrrhizae (*Gan Cao*), sesame oil, and beeswax as an external paste.

Dosage: 2-5g or 1-3 strips. When swallowed as a powder, take 0.6-1g each time. Externally, use a suitable amount.

Method of use: Commonly taken in powders and pills.

Cautions & contraindications: This medicinal is contraindicated in pregnant women or in those with blood vacuity tetany.

14

Orifice-opening medicinals

Medicinals whose main action is to open the orifices and arouse the spirit are called orifice-opening medicinals. Such medicinals have a relatively strong acrid, aromatic nature. Thus they have the effect of freeing the flow of the barriers and opening the orifices, penetrating and arousing the spirit. They are mainly suitable for use in heat falling into the pericardium or phlegm turbidity obstructing and confounding the heart orifices resulting in spirit clouding, delirious speech, fright epilepsy, wind stroke, and internal block repletion patterns marked by sudden fainting. Orifice-opening medicinals are not appropriate for vacuity desertion loss of consciousness. In addition, block patterns may be divided into the two types of cold and hot. Cold block should be treated by warm openers combined with ingredients which dispel cold and move the qi. Heat block should be treated by cool openers combined with ingredients which clear heat and resolve toxins.

Orifice-opening medicinals are for first aid emergency. They are branch treating ingredients. Therefore, they should only be used for a short period of time. Enduring administration is not appropriate so as to prevent consumption and discharge of the source qi. Furthermore, orifice-opening medicinals are acrid, aromatic ingredients. Their qi and flavor easily scatters and is lost. Therefore, they are mostly administered internally in the form of powders and pills.

Secretio Moschi Moschiferi (*She Xiang*)

Nature & flavor: Acrid and warm

Channel entry: Moves freely through all 12 channels

Functions: Opens the orifices and arouses the spirit, quickens the blood and scatters nodulations, stops pain, hastens birth

Indications:

1. Used for warm heat disease heat entering the pericardium spirit clouding, tetany reversal, wind stroke reversal, and fright epilepsy block conditions. If categorized as heat block, Secretio Moschi Moschiferi is commonly combined with Cornu Rhinocerotis[5] (*Xi Jiao*) and Calculus Bovis (*Niu Huang*) as in *Zhi Bao Dan* (Supreme Jewel Elixir). If categorized as cold block, Secretio Moschi Moschiferi is commonly combined with Styrax

Liquidus (*Su He Xiang*) and Flos Caryophylli (*Ding Xiang*) as in *Su He Xiang Wan* (Styrax Pills).

2. Used for sores and open sores swelling and toxins, Secretio Moschi Moschiferi is commonly combined with Realgar (*Xiong Huang*) and Resina Olibani (*Ru Xiang*) which can be both taken internally and applied externally, as in *Xing Xiao Wan* (Arouse & Disperse Pills). For the treatment of throat swelling and pain, Secretio Moschi Moschiferi is commonly combined with Calculus Bovis (*Niu Huang*), Realgar (*Xiong Huang*), and Borneolum (*Bing Pian*) as in *Liu Shen Wan* (Six Spirits Pills).

3. Used for heart and abdominal sudden or violent pain, traumatic injury stasis pain, and impediment conditions aching and pain. For the treatment of heart and abdominal aching and pain, Secretio Moschi Moschiferi can be combined with Radix Auklandiae Lappae (*Mu Xiang*) and Semen Pruni Persicae (*Tao Ren*). For the treatment of fall and strike detriment and damage, static blood, swelling, and pain, it can be combined with Lignum Sappan (*Su Mu*) and Resina Myrrhae (*Mo Yao*).

4. Used for concretions and conglomerations, blocked menstruation, a dead fetus within the abdomen, and non-descension of the placenta, Secretio Moschi Moschiferi is commonly combined with Rhizoma Sparganii (*San Leng*), Rhizoma Curcumae Zedoariae (*E Zhu*), and Cortex Cinnamomi Cassiae (*Rou Gui*).

Dosage: 0.06-0.1g. Externally, use a suitable amount.

Method of use: Only taken in pills and powders, this medicinal should never be decocted.

Cautions & contraindications: This medicinal is contraindicated in pregnant women.

Borneolum (*Bing Pian*)

Nature & flavor: Acrid, bitter, and slightly cold

Channel entry: Heart, liver, spleen, and lungs

Functions: Opens the orifices and arouses the spirit, clears heat and stops pain

Indications:

1. Used for wind stroke phlegm reversal, spirit clouding, and fright reversal, Borneolum is often combined with Secretio Moschi Moschiferi (*She Xiang*) as in *An Gong Niu Huang Wan* (Quiet the Palace Cow Bezoar Pills) and *Zhi Bao Dan* (Supreme Jewel Elixir).

2. Used for throat swelling and pain, sores in the mouth and on the tongue, red, swollen, painful eyes, and sores and open sores. For the treatment of throat swelling and pain, Borneolum can be combined with Borax (*Peng Sha*), Cinnabar (*Zhu Sha*), and refined Mirabilitum (*Xuan Ming Fen*). This is then called *Bing Peng San* (Borneol & Borax Powder). For the treatment of red, swollen, painful eyes, Borneolum can be combined with Rhizoma Coptidis Chinensis (*Huang Lian*) and Calamina (*Lu Gan Shi*) as in *Bo Yun San* (Setting Aside the Clouds Powder). In addition, Borneolum is used as an ingredient in many compound formulas for clearing heat and engendering muscle.

Dosage: 0.03-0.1g. Externally, use a suitable amount.

Method of use: Only used in pills and powders, this medicinal is never taken in decoction. For clearing heat and stopping pain, preventing putrefaction and dispersing swelling, this medicinal is usually used applied externally.

Rhizoma Acori Graminei (*Shi Chang Pu*)

Nature & flavor: Acrid, bitter, and warm

Channel entry: Heart, spleen, and stomach

Functions: Opens the orifices and calms the spirit, transforms dampness and harmonizes the stomach

Indications:

1. Used for damp turbidity confounding the clear orifices resulting in spirit will clouding and chaos, Rhizoma Acori Graminei is commonly combined with Tuber Curcumae (*Yu Jin*) and Rhizoma Pinelliae Ternatae (*Ban Xia*). Rhizoma Acori Graminei can also be used for withdrawal and torpid intelligence, in which case it is ground into powder, decocted in pig heart soup, and taken.

2. Used for heart qi insufficiency heart palpitations, insomnia, impaired memory, and tinnitus, Rhizoma Acori Graminei is commonly combined with Radix Polygalae Tenuifoliae (*Yuan Zhi*), Sclerotium Poriae Cocos (*Fu Ling*), Radix Panacis Ginseng (*Ren Shen*), and Dens Draconis (*Long Chi*) as in *An Shen Ding Zhi Wan* (Quiet the Spirit & Stabilize the Will Pills).

3. Used for damp obstructing the spleen and stomach chest oppression and abdominal distention, scanty eating and torpid intake, Rhizoma Acori Graminei can be combined with Pericarpium Citri Reticulatae (*Chen Pi*), Cortex Magnoliae Officinalis (*Hou Po*), and Rhizoma Pinelliae Ternatae (*Ban Xia*).

Dosage: 3-10g

Method of use: Decoct in water and administer internally.

Styrax Liquidus (*Su He Xiang*)

Nature & flavor: Acrid and warm

Channel entry: Heart and spleen

Functions: Opens the orifices and repels filth, scatters cold and stops pain

Indications:

1. Used for wind stroke phlegm reversal sudden fainting and syncope or withdrawal and epilepsy categorized as cold evils with phlegm turbidity blocking internally, Styrax Liquidus is commonly combined with Secretio Moschi Moschiferi (*She Xiang*), Flos Caryophylli (*Ding Xiang*), and Benzoin (*An Xi Xiang*) as in *Su He Xiang Wan* (Styrax Pills).

2. Used for chest and abdominal chilly pain, fullness, and oppression, Styrax Liquidus can be combined with Rhizoma Cyperi Rotundi (*Xiang Fu*), Rhizoma Corydalis Yanhusuo (*Yan Hu Suo*), Resina Olibani (*Ru Xiang*), and Resina Myrrhae (*Mo Yao*). For the treatment of chest impediment aching and pain, it can be combined with Lignum Santali Albi (*Tan Xiang*), Borneolum (*Bing Pian*), and Radix Auklandiae Lappae (*Mu Xiang*).

Nowadays, when this ingredient is used in combination with Borneolum (*Bing Pian*) in the treatment of the angina pectoris of coronary heart disease, it gets relatively good results.

Dosage: 0.3-1g

Method of use: Taken as pills and powders. This medicinal should not be decocted.

Cautions & contraindications: This medicinal should not be used for heat block conditions.

15

Supplementing & boosting medicinals

Medicinals which are able to supplement and boost the human body's qi, blood, yin, and yang insufficiency, raise the body's immunity, and therefore treat various types of vacuity weakness conditions are called supplementing and boosting medicinals. They are also called supplementing vacuity medicinals and supplementing and nourishing medicinals.

Vacuity patterns are divided into qi vacuity, yang vacuity, blood vacuity, and yin vacuity. Likewise, supplementing and boosting medicinals are also divided into those which supplement the qi, those which supplement yang, those which supplement the blood, and those which supplement yin. Because the human body's qi, blood, yin, and yang are all mutually interconnected, in yang vacuity, there is typically simultaneously qi vacuity, while qi vacuity may easily lead to yang vacuity. In yin vacuity, there is typically simultaneous blood vacuity, while blood vacuity easily leads to yin vacuity. Hence, it is common for qi and yang supplementing medicinals to be used together and for blood and yin supplementing medicinals to be used together. If there is a qi and blood insufficiency or a yin and yang dual vacuity existing at the same time, then it is necessary to supplement both the qi and blood or both the yin and yang.

It is not appropriate to use supplementing and boosting medicinals when replete evils have not yet been eliminated and the righteous qi is not vacuous in order to avoid interfering with the dispelling and elimination of replete evils and aggravating the disease condition. However, even if the disease evils have not yet been cleared, if the righteous qi is already vacuous, then one can combine evil-dispelling medicinals with supplementing and boosting medicinals. This is in order to increase and strengthen the immunity, support the righteous and dispel evils.

A. Qi-supplementing medicinals

Radix Panacis Ginseng (*Ren Shen*)

Nature & flavor: Sweet, slightly bitter, and level

Channel entry: Spleen, lungs, and heart

Functions: Greatly supplements the source qi, restores the pulse and secures desertion, supplements the spleen and boosts the lungs, engenders fluids and stops thirst, quiets the spirit and boosts the intelligence

Indications:

1. Used for qi vacuity on the verge of desertion. After great disease, enduring disease, great bleeding, or great vomiting or diarrhea, one may see the symptoms of qi shortness, lassitude of the spirit, and a minute pulse on the verge of expiry. This is a pattern of extreme vacuity on the verge of desertion. In such cases, Radix Panacis Ginseng can be used alone as a thick decoction in large doses. This is called *Du Shen Tang* (Solitary Ginseng Decoction). For qi desertion with simultaneous sweating, chilled limbs, and other such symptoms of perishing yang, Radix Panacis Ginseng can be combined with Radix Lateralis Praeparatus Aconiti Carmichaeli. This is then called *Shen Fu Tang* (Ginseng & Aconite Decoction).

2. Used for spleen vacuity conditions. For spleen qi insufficiency fatigue, lack of strength, devitalized eating and drinking, upper abdominal glomus and fullness, diarrhea, and various other symptoms due to qi vacuity bodily weakness, Radix Panacis Ginseng is commonly combined with Rhizoma Atractylodis Macrocephalae (*Bai Zhu*), Sclerotium Poriae Cocos (*Fu Ling*), and mix-fried Radix Glycyrrhizae (*Gan Cao*) as in *Si Jun Zi Tang* (Four Gentlemen Decoction).

3. Used for lung qi debility and vacuity. For lung qi vacuity coughing and panting, qi shortness, lack of strength, a vacuous pulse, and spontaneous perspiration, Radix Panacis Ginseng is often combined with Semen Juglandis Regiae (*Hu Tao Ren*), Fructus Schisandrae Chinensis (*Wu Wei Zi*), and Gecko (*Ge Jie*) as in *Ren Shen Hu Tao Tang* (Ginseng & Walnut Decoction) and *Ren Shen Ge Jie San* (Ginseng & Gecko Powder). For vacuity taxation cough with threads of blood within the phlegm, Radix Panacis Ginseng can be combined with Radix Asteris Tatarici (*Zi Wan*), Rhizoma Anemarrhenae Aspheloidis (*Zhi Mu*), and Gelatinum Corii Asini (*E Jiao*) as in *Zi Wan Tang* (Aster Decoction).

4. Used for fluid damage oral thirst and wasting and thirsting condition. For heat disease damaging both the qi and fluids with shortness of qi, oral thirst, profuse sweating, and a vacuous, minute, fine pulse, Radix Panacis Ginseng is commonly combined with Tuber Ophiopogonis Japonici (*Mai Men Dong*) and Fructus Schisandrae Chinensis (*Wu Wei Zi*). This is then called *Sheng Mai San* (Engender the Pulse Powder). In recent years, an injectable form of this prescription has be used for rescuing those in shock. For wasting and thirsting oral thirst and polyuria, Radix Panacis Ginseng is commonly combined with uncooked Radix Rehmanniae (*Sheng Di*), Tuber Ophiopogonis Japonici (*Mai Men Dong*), Radix Scrophulariae Ningpoensis (*Xuan Shen*), and Radix Trichosanthis Kirlowii (*Tian Hua Fen*).

5. Used for heart-spleen vacuity heart spirit restlessness, insomnia, profuse dreams, fright palpitations, impaired memory, bodily fatigue, and lack of strength, Radix Panacis Ginseng is commonly combined with Radix Angelicae Sinensis (*Dang Gui*), Semen Zizyphi

Spinosae (*Suan Zao Ren*), and Arillus Euphoriae Longanae (*Long Yan Rou*) as in *Gui Pi Tang* (Return the Spleen Decoction).

6. Used for qi and blood dual vacuity or blood vacuity conditions. For qi and blood dual vacuity, Radix Panacis Ginseng is commonly combined with uncooked Radix Rehmanniae (*Shu Di*) as in *Lian Yi Gao* (Dual Principle Paste). For blood vacuity, it can be combined with Radix Angelicae Sinensis (*Dang Gui*) and other blood-supplementing medicinals.

In addition, when Radix Panacis Ginseng is combined with yang-supplementing medicinals, it can be used for kidney vacuity impotence. In the treatment of bodily vacuity external contraction or for those with bodily vacuity who cannot endure attacking and precipitating formulas, Radix Panacis Ginseng can be incorporated in such formulas in order to increase and strengthen the power of disease resistance, support the righteous and dispel evils.

Dosage: 3-10g. When ground into powder and swallowed, take 1-2g each time. For rescuing from vacuity desertion, one can use doses as large as 15-30g, decocted and taken in divided doses.

Method of use: When taken in decoction, Radix Panacis Ginseng should be decocted alone over a slow fire and then mixed with the medicinal juice of the other decocted medicinals. It may also be ground into powder and swallowed.

Cautions & contraindications: Radix Panacis Ginseng is contraindicated in repletion patterns, heat patterns, and in cases where the righteous qi is not vacuous. It should not be combined with Radix Et Rhizoma Veratri (*Li Lu*), Feces Trogopterori Seu Pteromi (*Wu Ling Zhi*), and Fructus Gleditschiae Chinensis (*Zao Jiao*). When taking this medicinal, it is not appropriate to eat radish or drink tea in order to prevent any reduction in this medicinal's strength.

Radix Codonopsitis Pilosulae (*Dang Shen*)

Nature & flavor: Sweet and level

Channel entry: Spleen and lungs

Functions: Supplements the center and boosts the qi, engenders fluids and nourishes the blood

Indications:

1. Used for spleen vacuity conditions. For spleen qi insufficiency fatigue, lack of strength, scanty eating, loose stools, and various other symptoms due to qi vacuity and bodily

weakness, Radix Codonopsitis Pilosulae is commonly combined with Rhizoma Atractylodis Macrocephalae (*Bai Zhu*), Sclerotium Poriae Cocos (*Fu Ling*), and Radix Glycyrrhizae (*Gan Cao*). This ingredient's action is similar to that of Radix Panacis Ginseng (*Ren Shen*). In ordinary disease conditions, it can be used as a substitute for Radix Panacis Ginseng. However, its power to supplement the qi is weak. Therefore, for qi vacuity on the verge of desertion, it is not appropriate.

2. Used for lung qi debility and vacuity qi shortness, coughing, and panting, lack power to speak, and lowered and weak voice, Radix Codonopsitis Pilosulae is commonly combined with Radix Astragali Membranacei (*Huang Qi*) and Fructus Schisandrae Chinensis (*Wu Wei Zi*) as in *Bu Fei Tang* (Supplement the Lungs Decoction).

3. Used for heat disease dual damage to the qi and fluids with qi shortness and oral thirst, Radix Codonopsitis Pilosulae can be combined with Tuber Ophiopogonis Japonici (*Mai Men Dong*) and Fructus Schisandrae Chinensis (*Wu Wei Zi*).

4. Used for blood vacuity dizziness or a yellow facial complexion and superficial edema, Radix Codonopsitis Pilosulae can be combined with Radix Angelicae Sinensis (*Dang Gui*), cooked Radix Rehmanniae (*Shu Di*), Radix Albus Paeoniae Lactiflorae (*Bai Shao*), and Caulis Milletiae Seu Spatholobi (*Ji Xue Teng*).

In addition, this ingredient can also be added to those medicinals which resolve the exterior, attack, and precipitate when there is bodily vacuity with external affection of constipation and a righteous qi vacuity.

Dosage: 10-15g. In larger doses, up to 30g can be used.

Method of use: Decoct in water and administer internally or take in powders or pills.

Cautions & contraindications: This medicinal is not appropriate for use in those with heat patterns, yin vacuity yang hyperactivity patterns, or for those with center fullness evil repletion patterns.

Radix Astragali Membranacei (*Huang Qi*)

Nature & flavor: Sweet and warm

Channel entry: Spleen and lungs

Functions: Supplements the qi and upbears yang, boosts the defensive and secures the exterior, out-thrusts toxins and engenders muscle, disinhibits water and disperses swelling

Indications:

1. Used for spleen-lung qi vacuity and central qi downward fall conditions. For the treatment of qi vacuity and bodily weakness after disease with fatigue and lack of strength, Radix Astragali Membranacei is commonly combined with Radix Panacis Ginseng (*Ren Shen*) as in *Shen Qi Tang* (Ginseng & Astragalus Decoction). If there is simultaneous yang vacuity with fear of cold and profuse sweating, Radix Astragali Membranacei can be combined with Radix Lateralis Praeparatus Aconiti Carmichaeli (*Fu Zi*) as in *Qi Fu Gao* (Astragalus & Aconite Paste). For qi vacuity and blood debility, Radix Astragali Membranacei can be combined with Radix Angelicae Sinensis (*Dang Gui*). For spleen qi vacuity weakness with scanty eating and loose stools or diarrhea, Radix Astragali Membranacei can be combined with Rhizoma Atractylodis Macrocephalae (*Bai Zhu*). For central qi downward fall, prolapse of the internal viscera, uterine prolapse, and enduring diarrhea anal desertion, it can be combined with Radix Panacis Ginseng (*Ren Shen*), Rhizoma Atractylodis Macrocephalae (*Bai Zhu*), Rhizoma Cimicifugae (*Sheng Ma*), and Radix Bupleuri (*Chai Hu*) as in *Bu Zhong Yi Qi Tang* (Supplement the Center & Boost the Qi Decoction). For qi vacuity inability to manage, *i.e.*, contain, the blood hemafecia and flooding and leaking, Radix Astragali Membranacei can also be combined with Radix Panacis Ginseng (*Ren Shen*), Semen Zizyphi Spinosae (*Suan Zao Ren*), and Arillus Euphoriae Longanae (*Long Yan Rou*) as in *Gui Pi Tang* (Return the Spleen Decoction).

2. Used for qi vacuity and bodily weakness insecurity of the muscle exterior spontaneous perspiration and night sweats. For the treatment of bodily vacuity profuse sweating and easy catching of cold, Radix Astragali Membranacei is commonly combined with Rhizoma Atractylodis Macrocephalae (*Bai Zhu*) and Radix Ledebouriellae Divaricatae (*Fang Feng*) as in *Yu Ping Feng San* (Jade Windscreen Powder). It can also be combined with Concha Ostreae (*Mu Li*), Fructus Levis Tritici Aestivi (*Fu Xiao Mai*), and Radix Ephedrae (*Ma Huang Gen*) as in *Mu Li San* (Oyster Shell Powder). For night sweats, Radix Astragali Membranacei can be combined with uncooked Radix Rehmanniae (*Sheng Di*) and Cortex Phellodendri (*Huang Bai*) as in *Dang Gui Liu Huang Tang* (Dang Gui Six Yellows Decoction).

3. Used for qi and blood insufficiency resulting in welling and flat abscesses not rupturing or rupturing and then not constraining, *i.e.*, closing, for a long time. For the treatment of welling and flat abscesses not rupturing, Radix Astragali Membranacei is commonly combined with Squama Manitis Pentadactylis (*Chuan Shan Jia*), Radix Angelicae Sinensis (*Dang Gui*), and Spina Gleditschiae Chinensis (*Zao Jiao Ci*) as in *Tuo Nong San* (Out-thrust Pus Powder). For rupturing and then not constraining for a long time, Radix Astragali Membranacei can be combined with Radix Angelicae Sinensis (*Dang Gui*), Radix Panacis Ginseng (*Ren Shen*), and Cortex Cinnamomi Cassiae (*Rou Gui*) as in *Shi Quan Da Bu Tang* (Ten [Ingredients] Completely & Greatly Supplementing Decoction). For diabetes mellitus accompanied by welling abscess swelling and sores, uncooked Radix

Astragali Memebranacei can be combined with Radix Glycyrrhizae (*Gan Cao*) at a ratio of 6:1. These are ground into fine powder and 9g are taken each time, 2-3 times per day. Or these may be decocted in water and administered.

4. Used for qi vacuity loss of movement face and eye superficial edema, scanty urination, heart palpitations, and rapid breathing, *i.e.*, shortness of breath, Radix Astragali Membranacei should be combined with Radix Stephaniae Tetrandrae (*Han Fang Ji*) and Rhizoma Atractylodis Macrocephalae (*Bai Zhu*) as in *Fang Ji Huang Qi Tang* (Stephania & Astragalus Decoction). For chronic nephritis, use 15-30g or combine with Radix Codonopsitis Pilosulae (*Dang Shen*), decoct in water, and administer. This has the action of dispersing and eliminating proteinuria.

5. Used for qi vacuity blood stagnation numbness of the extremities and hemiplegia after a wind stroke with a clear spirit and weak pulse. For the former, Radix Astragali Membranacei can be combined with Ramulus Cinnamomi Cassiae (*Gui Zhi*) and Radix Albus Paeoniae Lactiflorae (*Bai Shao*) as in *Huang Qi Gui Zhi Wu Wu Tang* (Astragalus & Cinnamon Twig Five Materials Decoction). For the latter, Radix Astragali Membranacei is often combined with Radix Angelicae Sinensis (*Dang Gui*), Flos Carthami Tinctorii (*Hong Hua*), and Semen Pruni Persicae (*Tao Ren*) as in *Bu Yang Huan Wu Tang* (Supplement Yang & Restore the Five [Viscera] Decoction).

In addition, Radix Astragali Membranacei can also be combined with uncooked Radix Rehmanniae (*Sheng Di*), Tuber Ophiopogonis Japonici (*Mai Men Dong*), Radix Trichosanthis Kirlowii (*Tian Hua Fen*), and Radix Dioscoreae Oppositae (*Shan Yao*) for the treatment of wasting and thirsting condition.

Dosage: 10-15g or in larger doses up to 30-60g.

Method of use: Decoct in water and administer internally. For supplementing the qi and upbearing yang, one should use mix-fried. For other purposes, it should be used uncooked.

Cautions & contraindications: In cases of exterior repletion evil exuberance, qi stagnation damp obstruction, food accumulation collecting internally, yin vacuity yang hyperactivity, and the initial stage of welling and flat abscesses or if they have ruptured but there is enduring heat toxins which are still exuberant, Radix Astragali Membranacei should not be used. Use of excessively large doses of this medicinal can result in chest oppression and abdominal distention and scanty eating. In such cases, Radix Astragali Membranacei can be combined with qi-moving, stomach-opening medicinals such as Pericarpium Citri Reticulatae (*Chen Pi*) depending on the condition.

Rhizoma Atractylodis Macrocephalae (*Bai Zhu*)

Nature & flavor: Sweet, bitter, and warm

Channel entry: Spleen and stomach

Functions: Supplements the qi and fortifies the spleen, dries dampness and disinhibits water, stops sweating and quiets the fetus

Indications:

1. Used for spleen-stomach qi vacuity with loss of normalcy of movement and transformation resulting in scanty eating, loose stool, stomach duct and abdominal distention and fullness, fatigue, and lack of strength, Rhizoma Atractylodis Macrocephalae can be combined with Radix Panacis Ginseng (*Ren Shen*), Sclerotium Poriae Cocos (*Fu Ling*), and Radix Glycyrrhizae (*Gan Cao*) as in *Si Jun Zi Tang* (Four Gentlemen Decoction). For more severe vacuity cold with symptoms of stomach duct and abdominal chilly pain and diarrhea, Rhizoma Atractylodis Macrocephalae can be combined with Radix Codonopsitis Pilosulae (*Dang Shen*) and dry Rhizoma Zingiberis (*Gan Jiang*) as in *Li Zhong Tang* (Rectify the Center Decoction). For spleen vacuity with accumulation and stagnation, devitalized eating and drinking, and stomach duct and abdominal glomus and fullness, it can be combined with Fructus Immaturus Citri Aurantii (*Zhi Shi*) as in *Zhi Zhu Wan* (Aurantium & Atractylodes Pills).

2. Used for spleen vacuity loss of movement with water dampness collecting and retention, phlegm rheum, and water swelling. For phlegm rheum collecting and gathering with chest and rib-side fullness and oppression and dizziness, Rhizoma Atractylodis Macrocephalae can be combined with Ramulus Cinnamomi Cassiae (*Gui Zhi*), Sclerotium Poriae Cocos (*Fu Ling*), and mix-fried Radix Glycyrrhizae (*Gan Cao*). This is then called *Ling Gui Zhu Gan Tang* (Poria, Cinnamon, Atractylodes & Licorice Decoction). For water swelling, Rhizoma Atractylodis Macrocephalae can be combined with Sclerotium Poriae Cocos (*Fu Ling*), Rhizoma Alismatis (*Ze Xie*), and Ramulus Cinnamomi Cassiae (*Gui Zhi*) or with Radix Lateralis Praeparatus Aconiti Carmichaeli (*Fu Zi*) and dry Rhizoma Zingiberis (*Gan Jiang*) as in *Wu Ling San* (Five [Ingredients] Poria Powder) and *Zhen Wu Tang* (True Warrior Decoction) respectively.

3. Used for spleen vacuity qi weakness and insecurity of the muscle exterior sweating, Rhizoma Atractylodis Macrocephalae can be combined with Radix Astragali Membranacei (*Huang Qi*), and Fructus Levis Tritici Aestivi (*Fu Xiao Mai*).

4. Used for spleen vacuity qi weakness and fetal stirring restlessness. If there is internal heat, Rhizoma Atractylodis Macrocephalae can be combined with Radix Scutellariae

Baicalensis (*Huang Qin*). If there is simultaneous qi stagnation abdominal distention, it can be combined with Caulis Perillae Frutescentis (*Su Gen*) and Fructus Amomi (*Sha Ren*). For severe qi vacuity and lack of strength, Rhizoma Atractylodis Macrocephalae can be combined with Radix Codonopsitis Pilosulae (*Dang Shen*), Sclerotium Poriae Cocos (*Fu Ling*), and Radix Glycyrrhizae (*Gan Cao*). If there is simultaneous blood vacuity dizziness and heart fluster, *i.e.*, palpitations, it can be combined with cooked Radix Rehmanniae (*Shu Di*), Radix Angelicae Sinensis (*Dang Gui*), and Radix Albus Paeoniae Lactiflorae (*Bai Shao*). For a relatively severe condition of low back aching and abdominal pain, Rhizoma Atractylodis Macrocephalae can be combined with Cortex Eucommiae Ulmoidis (*Du Zhong*), Gelatinum Corii Asini (*E Jiao*), and Radix Dipsaci (*Xu Duan*).

Dosage: 6-15g

Method of use: Decoct in water or take in powders or pills. For drying dampness and disinhibiting water, one should use uncooked. For supplementing the qi and fortifying the spleen, one should use bran stir-fried. For fortifying the spleen and stopping diarrhea, one should use earth stir-fried or stir-fried till scorched.

Cautions & contraindications: This medicinal should not be used in those with yin vacuity internal heat or fluid and humor consumption, dryness, and thirst. Due to its dry nature, it easily damages yin.

Radix Dioscoreae Oppositae (*Shan Yao*)

Nature & flavor: Sweet and level

Channel entry: Spleen, lungs, and kidneys

Functions: Supplements the spleen and nourishes the stomach, engenders fluids and boosts the lungs, supplements the kidneys and secures the essence

Indications:

1. Used for spleen-stomach vacuity weakness, scanty eating, bodily fatigue, and loose stools or diarrhea, Radix Dioscoreae Oppositae is commonly combined with Radix Panacis Ginseng (*Ren Shen*), Rhizoma Atractylodis Macrocephalae (*Bai Zhu*), and Sclerotium Poriae Cocos (*Fu Ling*) as in *Shen Ling Bai Zhu San* (Ginseng, Poria & Atractylodes Powder).

2. Used for lung vacuity panting and cough, Radix Dioscoreae Oppositae is commonly combined with Radix Codonopsitis Pilosulae (*Dang Shen*), Tuber Ophiopogonis Japonici (*Mai Dong*), and Fructus Schisandrae Chinensis (*Wu Wei Zi*).

3. Used for kidney vacuity seminal emission, abnormal vaginal discharge, or frequent urination. For kidney vacuity seminal emission, Radix Dioscoreae Oppositae can be combined with cooked Radix Rehmanniae (*Shu Di*) and Fructus Corni Officinalis (*Shan Zhu Yu*) as in *Liu Wei Di Huang Wan* (Six Flavors Rehmannia Pills). For frequent urination, it can be combined with Fructus Alpiniae Oxyphyllae (*Yi Zhi Ren*) and Radix Linderae Strychnifoliae (*Wu Yao*) as in *Suo Quan Wan* (Stream-reducing Pills). For women's excessively profuse vaginal discharge categorized as spleen vacuity with dampness, Radix Dioscoreae Oppositae is commonly combined with Radix Codonopsitis Pilosulae (*Dang Shen*), Rhizoma Atractylodis Macrocephalae (*Bai Zhu*), and Semen Plantaginis (*Che Qian Zi*). For yellow vaginal discharge with damp heat, it should be combined with Cortex Phellodendri (*Huang Bai*). For kidney vacuity not securing, it can be combined with cooked Radix Rehmanniae (*Shu Di*), Fructus Corni Officinalis (*Shan Zhu Yu*), and Semen Cuscutae Chinensis (*Tu Si Zi*).

4. Used for wasting and thirsting or yin vacuity fluid debility, vexatious heat, and oral thirst. For the treatment of mild wasting and thirsting, Radix Dioscoreae Oppositae can be decocted and drunk as a beverage tea, 250g per day, for a prolonged period of time. It can also be combined with Radix Astragali Membranacei (*Huang Qi*), Radix Puerariae (*Ge Gen*), Radix Trichosanthis Kirlowii (*Tian Hua Fen*), and Rhizoma Anemarrhenae Aspheloidis (*Zhi Mu*) as in *Yu Ye Tang* (Jade Humor Decoction). For the treatment of fluid debility oral thirst, it can be combined with Tuber Ophiopogonis Japonici (*Mai Men Dong*) and Rhizoma Polygonati Odorati (*Yu Zhu*).

Dosage: 10-30g, and in larger doses of 60-120g. When taken as a ground powder, 6-10g each time.

Method of use: Decoct in water and administer internally. For nourishing yin and engendering fluids, use uncooked. For fortifying the spleen and stopping diarrhea, use bran stir-fried.

Cautions & contraindications: This medicinal should not be used in those with damp exuberance center fullness or chest and abdominal fullness and oppression.

Radix Glycyrrhizae (*Gan Cao*)

Nature & flavor: Sweet and level

Channel entry: Heart, lungs, spleen, and stomach

Functions: Supplements the spleen and boosts the qi, dispels phlegm and stops cough, clears heat and resolves toxins, relaxes cramping and stops pain, regulates and harmonizes other medicinals' natures.

Indications:

1. Used for spleen-stomach qi vacuity, qi shortness, lack of strength, scanty eating, and loose stools, Radix Glycyrrhizae is commonly combined with Radix Codonopsitis Pilosulae (*Dang Shen*), Rhizoma Atractylodis Macrocephalae (*Bai Zhu*) as an adjuvant medicinal as in *Si Jun Zi Tang* (Four Gentlemen Decoction). For qi vacuity and scanty blood, heart palpitations, spontaneous perspiration, and a bound or regulary intermittent pulse, Radix Glycyrrhizae is often combined with uncooked Radix Rehmanniae (*Sheng Di*), Radix Codonopsitis Pilosulae (*Dang Shen*), Tuber Ophiopogonis Japonici (*Mai Dong*), and Ramulus Cinnamomi Cassiae (*Gui Zhi*) as in *Zhi Gan Cao Tang* (Mix-fried Licorice Decoction).

2. Used for cough and qi panting. For wind heat cough, Radix Glycyrrhizae can be combined with Radix Platycodi Grandiflori (*Jie Geng*), Fructus Arctii Lappae (*Niu Xi*), Radix Peucedani (*Qian Hu*), and Folium Mori Albi (*Sang Ye*). For wind cold cough, it can be combined with Herba Ephedrae (*Ma Huang*), and Semen Pruni Armeniacae (*Xing Ren*) as in *San Ao Tang* (Three Rough & Ready [Ingredients] Decoction). For lung heat coughing and panting, Radix Glycyrrhizae can be combined with uncooked Gypsum Fibrosum (*Shi Gao*), Herba Ephedrae (*Ma Huang*), and Semen Pruni Armeniacae (*Xing Ren*) as in *Ma Xing Shi Gan Tang* (Ephedra, Armeniaca, Gypsum & Licorice Decoction).

3. Used for sores and open sore swelling and toxins, throat swelling and pain, and poisoning due to foods and medicinals. For sores and open sores swelling and toxins, Radix Glycyrrhizae can be combined with Flos Lonicerae Japonicae (*Jin Yin Hua*) and Fructus Forsythiae Suspensae (*Lian Qiao*). For throat swelling and pain, it is commonly combined with Radix Platycodi Grandiflori (*Jie Geng*) as in *Jie Geng Tang* (Platycodon Decoction). For poisoning due to foods and medicinals, Radix Glycyrrhizae can be combined with Semen Phaseoli Munginis (*Lu Dou*) or Radix Ledebouriellae Divaricatae (*Fang Feng*) decocted in water and administered.

4. Used for stomach duct and abdominal as well as sinew vessel spasm, contraction, aching, and pain. For stomach duct and abdominal aching and pain, Radix Glycyrrhizae

is commonly combined with Ramulus Cinnamomi Cassiae (*Gui Zhi*), Radix Paeoniae Lactiflorae (*Shao Yao*), and Maltose (*Yi Tang*) as in *Xiao Jian Zhong Tang* (Minor Fortify the Center Decoction). For spasms and contractions of the four limbs, aching, and pain, Radix Glycyrrhizae is commonly combined with Radix Paeoniae Lactiflorae (*Shao Yao*). This is then called *Shao Yao Gan Cao Tang* (Peony & Licorice Decoction).

In addition, when Radix Glycyrrhizae is used in compound formulas, it can reduce or moderate and harmonize the preponderant natures or toxicity of other medicinal substances. At the same time, it regulates and harmonizes the actions of other medicinals in a formula.

Dosage: 3-6g. As the main medicinal in a formula, it can be used from 10-30g.

Method of use: Decoct in water and administer internally. This medicinal should be used uncooked when entered with clearing and draining medicinals. It should be used honey mix-fried when entered with supplementing and boosting medicinals.

Cautions & contraindications: Radix Glycyrrhizae is contraindicated in case of damp exuberance center fullness and vomiting and spitting. It should not be combined with Radix Euphorbiae Seu Knoxiae (*Da Ji*), Radix Euphorbiae Kansui (*Gan Sui*), or Flos Daphnes Genkwae (*Yuan Hua*). Enduring administration of relatively large doses easily leads to the arising of water swelling. Pay timely attention to this.

Fructus Zizyphi Jujubae (*Da Zao*)

Nature & flavor: Sweet and slightly warm

Channel entry: Spleen, stomach, heart, and liver

Functions: Supplements the center and boosts the qi, nourishes the blood and quiets the spirit, moderates and harmonizes the natures of other medicinals

Indications:

1. Used for spleen vacuity scanty eating, lack of strength, and loose stools, Fructus Zizyphi Jujubae is commonly combined with Radix Codonopsitis Pilosulae (*Dang Shen*), Radix Astragali Membranacei (*Huang Qi*), and Rhizoma Atractylodis Macrocephalae (*Bai Zhu*) as in *Gui Pi Tang* (Return the Spleen Decoction).

2. Used for qi and blood dual vacuity, Fructus Zizyphi Jujubae is commonly combined with Radix Codonopsitis Pilosulae (*Dang Shen*), Radix Angelicae Sinensis (*Dang Gui*), and Radix Glycyrrhizae (*Gan Cao*) as in *Ba Zhen Tang* (Eight Pearls Decoction).

3. Used for visceral agitation, Fructus Zizyphi Jujubae is commonly combined with Radix Glycyrrhizae (*Gan Cao*) and Fructus Levis Tritici Aestivi (*Fu Xiao Mai*) as in *Gan Mai Da Zao Tang* (Licorice, Wheat & Red Dates Decoction).

Dosage: 3-10 fruits. In larger doses, it can be used up to 30-60g.

Method of use: Decoct in water and administer internally.

Cautions & contraindications: This medicinal is able to strengthen dampness. Therefore, it is not appropriate to use in case of damp obstruction abdominal distention, fullness, and oppression.

B. Yang-supplementing medicinals

Cornu Parvum Cervi (*Lu Rong*)

Nature & flavor: Sweet, salty, and warm

Channel entry: Liver and kidneys

Functions: Supplements kidney yang, boosts the essence and blood, strengthen the sinews and bones

Indications:

1. Used for kidney yang insufficiency, essence blood debility and vacuity fear of cold, chilled limbs, impotence, slippery essence, uterine chill infertility, frequent, numerous urination, low back and knee aching and pain, dizziness, tinnitus, and essence spirit listlessness, Cornu Parvum Cervi can be used alone ground into powder and taken or combined with Radix Panacis Ginseng (*Ren Shen*), cooked Radix Rehmanniae (*Shu Di*), and Fructus Lycii Chinensis (*Gou Qi Zi*) as in *Shen Rong Gu Ben Wan* (Ginseng & Deer Antler Secure the Root Pills).

2. Used for liver-kidney insufficiency, sinew bone lack of strength, and children's maldevelopment, slowness walking, slowness teething, non-closure of the fontanels, etc., Cornu Parvum Cervi is commonly combined with uncooked Radix Rehmanniae (*Shu Di*),

Radix Dioscoreae Oppositae (*Shan Yao*), and Fructus Corni Officinalis (*Shan Zhu Yu*) as in *Jia Wei Di Huang Wan* (Added Flavors Rehmannia Pills).

3. Used for women's *chong* and *ren* vacuity cold flooding and leaking and *dai mai* not securing increased, profuse abnormal vaginal discharge. For the former, Cornu Parvum Cervi can be combined with Gelatinum Corii Asini (*E Jiao*) and Os Sepiae Seu Sepiellae (*Wu Zei Gu*) as in *Lu Rong San* (Deer Antler Powder). For the latter, it can be combined with Rhizoma Cibotii Barometsis (*Gou Ji*) and Radix Ampelosis (*Bai Lian*).

In addition, Cornu Parvum Cervi is effective for yin flat abscesses falling inward and not arising or sores which have ruptured and not constrained or closed due to its warming, supplementing, and out-thrusting sores.

Dosage: 1-3g. 0.5-1g each time when swallowed as a powder.

Method of use: Grind into powder and take three times per day, or administer in pills and powders.

Cautions & contraindications: This ingredient's nature is warm. Therefore, it is contraindicated in yin vacuity yang hyperactivity, blood heat, stomach fire hyperactivity and exuberance, phlegm heat cough, and eternal affection disease.

Herba Epimedii (*Yin Yang Huo*)

Nature & flavor: Acrid, sweet, and warm

Channel entry: Liver and kidneys

Functions: Supplements the kidneys and invigorates yang, dispels wind and eliminates dampness

Indications:

1. Used for kidney vacuity impotence, low back and knee lack of strength, frequent urination, and female infertility, Herba Epimedii can be used alone, soaked in alcohol, and administered as a tincture, or it may be combined with cooked Radix Rehmanniae (*Shu Di*), Fructus Corni Officinalis (*Shan Zhu Yu*), Rhizoma Cucurliginis Orchioidis (*Xian Mao*), and Fructus Lycii Chinensis (*Gou Qi Zi*).

2. Used for wind cold damp impediment, sinew bone contracture, and numbness of the hands and feet, Herba Epimedii can be combined with Radix Clematidis Chinensis (*Wei

Ling Xian) and Fructus Xanthii Sibirici (*Cang Er Zi*) as in *Xian Ling Pi San* (Epimedium Powder).

In addition, Herba Epimedii can be combined with Rhizoma Curculiginis Orchioidis (*Xian Mao*) and Radix Morindae Officinalis (*Ba Ji Tian*) as in *Er Xian Tang* (Two Immortals Decoction) for climacteric high blood pressure. It may be combined with Fructus Psoraleae Corylifoliae (*Bu Gu Zhi*), Semen Juglandis Regiae (*Hu Tao Ren*), and Fructus Schisandrae Chinensis (*Wu Wei Zi*) for yang vacuity panting and coughing.

Dosage: 6-12g

Method of use: Decoct in water and administer internally. It may also be soaked in alcohol, simmered into paste. Or taken as pills or powders.

Cautions & contraindications: It is not appropriate to administer this medicinal in cases of yin vacuity fire effulgence. Due to its drying nature, it is able to damage yin and invigorate fire.

Rhizoma Curculiginis Orchioidis (*Xian Mao*)

Nature & flavor: Acrid and hot. Has small toxins.

Channel entry: Kidneys and liver

Functions: Supplements kidney yang, strengthens the sinews and bones, dispels cold and dampness

Indications:

1. Used for kidney yang vacuity low back and knee chill and pain, lack of sexual desire, cold feet, impotence, frequent urination, especially at night, and seminal emission, Rhizoma Curculiginis Orchioidis is commonly combined with Herba Epimedii (*Yin Yang Huo*) and Radix Morindae Officinalis (*Ba Ji Tian*) as in *Er Xian Tang* (Two Immortals Decoction).

2. Used for cold damp impediment pain and chill in the low back and legs, Rhizoma Curculiginis Orchioidis can be combined with Herba Asari Cum Radice (*Xi Xin*).

Dosage: 3-10g

Method of use: Decoct in water and administer internally.

Cautions & contraindications: One should not administer this supplementing medicinal for too long a time. Its use is contraindicated in case of yin vacuity fire effulgence or in those with a yang hyperactivity body.

Cortex Eucommiae Ulmoidis (*Du Zhong*)

Nature & flavor: Sweet and warm

Channel entry: Liver and kidneys

Functions: Supplements the liver and kidneys, strengthens the sinews and bones, quiets the fetus

Indications:

1. Used for liver-kidney insufficiency low back and knee aching and pain, sinew and bone lack of strength, impotence, and frequent urination. For the former, Cortex Eucommiae Ulmoidis is commonly combined with Fructus Psoraleae Corylifoliae (*Bu Gu Zhi*) as in *Qing E Wan* (Young Maid Pills). For the latter, it can be combined with Fructus Corni Officinalis (*Shan Zhu Yu*), Semen Cuscutae Chinensis (*Tu Si Zi*), and cooked Radix Rehmanniae (*Shu Di*).

2. Used for women's flooding and leaking or bodily vacuity during pregnancy fetal stirring or fetal leakage, Cortex Eucommiae Ulmoidis is commonly combined with Radix Dipsaci (*Xu Duan*) and Fructus Zizyphi Jujubae (*Da Zao*) as in *Du Zhong Wan* (Eucommia Pills). Or it can be combined with other supplementing, boosting, and securing the menses medicinals.

In addition, Cortex Eucommiae Ulmoidis can be used in the treatment of high blood pressure accompanied by kidney vacuity symptoms. In that case, it can be combined with Ramulus Loranthi Seu Visci (*Sang Ji Sheng*), Radix Achyranthis Bidentatae (*Niu Xi*), and Spica Prunellae Vulgaris (*Xia Ku Cao*).

Dosage: 10-15g

Method of use: Decoct in water and administer internally. Stir-fried Cortex Eucommiae Ulmoidis gets better therapeutic effects than uncooked.

Cautions & contraindications: It is not appropriate to use this medicinal in yin vacuity fire effulgence cases.

Radix Dipsaci (*Xu Duan*)

Nature & flavor: Bitter, sweet, acrid, and slightly warm

Channel entry: Liver and kidneys

Functions: Supplements the liver and kidneys, strengthens the sinews and bones, connect broken bones, and stops flooding and leaking

Indications:

1. Used for low back and leg pain and flaccidity due to liver-kidney yang vacuity or damp cold impediment as well as fetal stirring restlessness, Radix Dipsaci is commonly combined with Cortex Eucommiae Ulmoidis (*Du Zhong*).

2. Used for women's flooding and leaking due to vacuity cold, Radix Dipsaci can be combined with Folium Artemisiae Argyii (*Ai Ye*) and Radix Astragali Membranacei (*Huang Qi*).

Dosage: 10-15g

Method of administration: Decoct in water and administer internally.

Fructus Psoraleae Corylifoliae (*Bu Gu Zhi*)

Nature & flavor: Acrid, bitter, and warm

Channel entry: Kidneys and spleen

Functions: Supplements the kidneys and invigorates yang, secures the essence and reduces urine, warms the spleen and stops diarrhea

Indications:

1. Used for kidney vacuity impotence and seminal emission, low back and knee chilly pain, frequent urination, and enuresis. For the treatment of kidney vacuity low back pain, Fructus Psoraleae Corylifoliae can be combined with Cortex Eucommiae Ulmoidis (*Du Zhong*) and Semen Juglandis Regiae (*Hu Tao Ren*) as in *Qing E Wan* (Young Maid Pills). For the treatment of impotence and seminal emission, Fructus Psoraleae Corylifoliae is commonly combined with Semen Cuscutae Chinensis (*Tu Si Zi*) and Semen Juglandis Regiae (*Hu Tao Ren*) as in *Bu Gu Zhi Wan* (Psoralea Pills). For the treatment of frequent

urination and enuresis, it can be combined with Fructus Foeniculi Vulgaris (*Xiao Hui Xiang*) as in *Bo Gu Zhi Wan* (Psoralea Pills).[8]

2. Used for spleen-kidney yang vacuity fifth watch diarrhea, Fructus Psoraleae Corylifoliae is commonly combined with Semen Myristicae Fragrantis (*Rou Dou Kou*), Fructus Schisandrae Chinensis (*Wu Wei Zi*), and Fructus Evodiae Rutecarpae (*Wu Zhu Yu*). This is called *Si Shen Wan* (Four Spirits Pills).

In addition, when made into an alcohol tincture for external use, Fructus Psoraleae Corylifoliae can treat white patch wind and alopecia areata.

Dosage: 5-10g

Method of use: Decoct in water and administer internally or take in powders or pills.

Cautions & contraindications: Administration of the medicinal is contraindicated in yin vacuity fire effulgence and constipation.

Herba Cistanchis Deserticolae (*Rou Cong Rong*)

Nature & flavor: Sweet, salty, and warm

Channel entry: Kidneys and large intestine

Functions: Supplements the kidneys and invigorates yang, boosts the essence and blood, moistens the intestines and frees the flow of the stool

Indications:

1. Used for kidney vacuity impotence, low back and knee chilly pain, and female infertility. For the treatment of impotence, Herba Cistanchis Deserticolae is commonly combined with cooked Radix Rehmanniae (*Shu Di*), Semen Cuscutae Chinensis (*Tu Si Zi*), and Fructus Schisandrae Chinensis (*Wu Wei Zi*) as in *Rou Cong Rong Wan* (Cistanches Pills). For the treatment of low back and knee chilly pain and sinew and bone lack of strength, it is often combined with Radix Morindae Officinalis (*Ba Ji Tian*), Rhizoma Dioscoreae Hypoglaucae (*Bie Xie*), and Cortex Eucommiae Ulmoidis (*Du Zhong*) as in *Jin Gang Wan* (Metal Strength Pills). For the treatment of female infertility, Herba Cistanchis Deserticolae is combined with medicinals which supplement and boost the essence and

---

[8] In Chinese, Psoralea has two different names, one romanized as *Bu Gu Zhi*, the other as *Bo Gu Zhi*.

blood, such as Gelatinum Cornu Cervi (*Lu Jiao Jiao*), Radix Angelicae Sinensis (*Dang Gui*), and Placenta Hominis (*Zi He Che*).

2. Used for dry intestine constipation in the elderly and in those with bodily vacuity, Herba Cistanchis Deserticolae is commonly combined with Semen Cannabis Sativae (*Huo Ma Ren*) and Lignum Aquilariae Agallochae (*Chen Xiang*) as in *Run Chang Wan* (Moisten the Intestines Pills). For blood vacuity fluid debility, it can be combined with medicinals which engender fluids and nourish the blood, such as uncooked Radix Rehmanniae (*Sheng Di*) and Radix Angelicae Sinensis (*Dang Gui*).

Dosage: 10-20g. One can use larger doses up to 30g.

Method of use: Decoct in water and administer internally.

Cautions & contraindications: This medicinal should not be administered to those with yin vacuity fire effulgence, spleen vacuity loose stools, or replete heat constipation.

Semen Cuscutae Chinensis (*Tu Si Zi*)

Nature & flavor: Sweet, acrid, and warm

Channel entry: Liver and kidneys

Functions: Enriches and supplements the liver and kidneys, secures the essence and reduces urination, quiets the fetus, brightens the eyes, and stops diarrhea

Indications:

1. Used for spleen-kidney dual vacuity diarrhea and abnormal vaginal discharge, Semen Cuscutae Chinensis is commonly combined with Radix Dioscoreae Oppositae (*Shan Yao*). Add Fructus Psoraleae Corylifoliae (*Bu Gu Zhi*) and Fructus Corni Officinalis (*Shan Zhu Yu*) for premature ejaculation and seminal emission.

2. Used for fetal stirring restlessness, Semen Cuscutae Chinensis is commonly combined with Radix Dipsaci (*Xu Duan*), Cortex Eucommiae Ulmoidis (*Du Zhong*), and Ramulus Loranthi Seu Visci (*Sang Ji Sheng*).

3. Used for blurred vision and decreased visual acuity, Semen Cuscutae Chinensis can be combined with Semen Plantaginis (*Che Qian Zi*), Fructus Lycii Chinensis (*Gou Qi Zi*), and Fructus Ligustri Lucidi (*Nu Zhen Zi*).

4. Used for female infertility, Semen Cuscutae Chinensis is commonly combined with Fructus Lycii Chinensis (*Gou Qi Zi*), Fructus Rubi Chingii (*Fu Pen Zi*), and Fructus Schisandrae Chinensis (*Wu Wei Zi*).

Dosage: 10-15g

Method of use: Decoct in water and administer internally.

Cautions & contraindications: This medicinal is contraindicated in yin vacuity fire effulgence and intestinal dryness and binding.

Radix Morindae Officinalis (*Ba Ji Tian*)

Nature & flavor: Acrid, sweet, and slightly warm

Channel entry: Liver and kidneys

Functions: Supplements kidney yang, strengthens the sinews and bones, and dispels wind dampness

Indications:

1. Used for impotence and seminal emission, Radix Morindae Officinalis is commonly combined with Semen Cuscutae Chinensis (*Tu Si Zi*) and Herba Cistanchis Deserticolae (*Rou Cong Rong*).

2. Used for low back and knee soreness and pain due to kidney yang vacuity or cold damp impediment, sinew and bone wilting and flaccidity, Radix Morindae Officinalis can be combined with Cortex Eucommiae Ulmoidis (*Du Zhong*), Radix Dipsaci (*Xu Duan*), and Radix Achyranthis Bidentatae (*Niu Xi*).

Dosage: 6-10g

Method of use: Decoct in water and administer internally.

Cautions & contraindications: This medicinal is contraindicated in cases of yin vacuity fire effulgence, dry mouth and parched tongue, and inhibited urination.

Semen Juglandis Regiae (*Hu Tao Ren*)

Nature & flavor: Sweet and warm

Channel entry: Kidneys, lungs, and large intestine

Functions: Supplements the kidneys, warms the lungs, and moistens the intestines

Indications:

1. Used for low back and knee soreness and flaccidity due to kidney vacuity, Semen Juglandis Regiae can be combined with Cortex Eucommiae Ulmoidis (*Du Zhong*) and Fructus Psoraleae Corylifoliae (*Bu Gu Zhi*).

2. Used for vacuity cold panting and coughing, Semen Juglandis Regiae can be combined with Radix Panacis Ginseng (*Ren Shen*) and Gecko (*Ge Jie*).

3. Used for fluid dryness constipation, Semen Juglandis Regiae can be combined with Herba Cistanchis Deserticolae (*Rou Cong Rong*) and Semen Cannabis Sativae (*Huo Ma Ren*).

Dosage: 10-30g

Method of use: Decoct in water and administer internally.

Cautions & contraindications: This medicinal is contraindicated in cases of phlegm fire or hot cough or in those with loose stools or diarrhea.

Herba Cynomorii Songarici (*Suo Yang*)

Nature & flavor: Sweet and warm

Channel entry: Liver and kidneys

Functions: Supplements kidney yang, boosts the essence and blood, moistens the intestines and frees the flow of the stool

Indications:

1. Used for low back and knee wilting and flaccidity, Herba Cynomorii Songarici can be combined with cooked Radix Rehmanniae (*Shu Di*) and Radix Achyranthis Bidentatae (*Niu Xi*).

2. Used for urinary incontinence, frequent urination, and slippery essence, Herba Cynomorii Songarici can be combined with Ootheca Mantidis (*Sang Piao Xiao*).

3. Used for blood vacuity fluid dryness constipation, Herba Cynomorii Songarici can be used as a cheaper substitute for Herba Cistanchis Deserticolae (*Rou Cong Rong*).

Dosage: 4.5-10g

Method of use: Decoct in water and administer internally.

Cautions & contraindications: This medicinal is contraindicated in those with loose stools or diarrhea.

Gecko (*Ge Jie*)

Nature & flavor: Salty and level. Has small toxins.

Channel entry: Lungs and kidneys

Functions: Supplements the lungs and boosts the kidneys, grasps or absorbs the qi and stabilizes panting, invigorates yang and boosts the essence

Indications:

1. Used for vacuity panting and rapid breathing, Gecko is commonly combined with Radix Panacis Ginseng (*Ren Shen*), mix-fried Radix Glycyrrhizae (*Gan Cao*), Semen Pruni Armeniacae (*Xing Ren*), and Cortex Radicis Mori Albi (*Sang Bai Pi*) as in *Ren Shen Ge Jie San* (Ginseng & Gecko Powder).

2. Used for taxation cough and coughing of blood, Gecko can be combined with uncooked Radix Rehmanniae (*Sheng Di*).

3. Used for impotence and seminal emission, Gecko can be combined with Cornu Parvum Cervi (*Lu Rong*), Cortex Eucommiae Ulmoidis (*Du Zhong*), and Radix Panacis Ginseng (*Ren Shen*) as in *Ge Jie Bu Shen Wan* (Gecko Supplement the Kidneys Pills).

Dosage: 3-6g. Take 1-1.5g each time when swallowed as a powder.

Method of use: Decoct in water and administer internally, take in powders and pills, or soak in alcohol and take as a tincture.

Rhizoma Cibotii Barometsis (*Gou Ji*)

Nature & flavor: Bitter, sweet, and warm

Channel entry: Liver and kidneys

Functions: Supplements the liver and kidneys, strengthens the lower and upper back, dispels wind dampness

Indications:

1. Used for lower and upper back soreness and flaccidity and lower extremity lack of strength, Rhizoma Cibotii Barometsis can be combined with Cortex Eucommiae Ulmoidis (*Du Zhong*) and Radix Acyranthis Bidentatae (*Niu Xi*).

2. Used for wind damp impediment pain, especially in the low back, Rhizoma Cibotii Barometsis can be combined with Ramulus Cinnamomi Cassiae (*Gui Zhi*) and Radix Gentianae Macrophyllae (*Qin Jiao*).

Dosage: 6-12g

Method of use: Decoct in water and administer internally.

Placenta Hominis (*Zi He Che*)

Nature & flavor: Sweet, salty, and warm

Channel entry: Lungs, liver, and kidneys

Functions: Warms the kidneys and supplements the essence, boosts the qi and nourishes the blood

Indications:

1. Used for vacuity taxation emaciation, bone-steaming, and night sweats, Placenta Hominis can be combined with Radix Polygoni Multiflori (*He Shou Wu*), Fructus Schisandrae Chinensis (*Wu Wei Zi*), and Radix Astragali Membranacei (*Huang Qi*) as in *Shen Jing Shuai Rou Wan* (Neurasthenia Pills) or with Tuber Ophiopogonis Japonici (*Mai Men Dong*), cooked Radix Rehmanniae (*Shu Di*), Cortex Phellodendri (*Huang Bai*), and Plastrum Testudinis (*Gui Ban*) as in *He Che Da Zao Wan* (Placenta Greatly Building Pills).

2. Used for coughing and qi panting, Placenta Hominis can be combined with Fructus Schisandrae Chinensis (*Wu Wei Zi*) and Tuber Ophiopogonis Japonici (*Mai Men Dong*).

3. Used for infertility and scanty lactation, it can be combined with cooked Radix Rehmanniae (*Shu Di*), Radix Angelicae Sinensis (*Dang Gui*), Radix Albus Paeoniae Lactiflorae (*Bai Shao*), Radix Astragali Membranacei (*Huang Qi*), and Radix Codonopsitis Pilosulae (*Dang Shen*).

Dosage: 1.5-3g ground into powder and swallowed or taken in pills

C. Blood-supplementing medicinals

Radix Angelicae Sinensis (*Dang Gui*)

Nature & flavor: Sweet, acrid, bitter, and warm

Channel entry: Liver, heart, and spleen

Functions: Supplements the blood, quickens the blood, stops pain, moistens the intestines

Indications:

1. Used for blood vacuity sallow yellow facial complexion, pale lips and tongue, dizziness, heart palpitations, and somber white fingernails, Radix Angelicae Sinensis is commonly combined with Radix Astragali Membranacei (*Huang Qi*) as in *Dang Gui Bu Xue Tang* (Dang Gui Supplement the Blood Decoction).

2. Used for menstrual irregularity, blocked menstruation, and painful menstruation. If these are due to blood vacuity, Radix Angelicae Sinensis is commonly combined with cooked Radix Rehmanniae (*Shu Di*), Radix Albus Paeoniae Lactiflorae (*Bai Shao*), and Gelatinum Corii Asini (*E Jiao*) as in *Si Wu Tang* (Four Materials Decoction) and *Jiao Ai Tang* (Donkey Skin Glue & Mugwort Decoction). If due to blood stasis, it is commonly combined with Radix Ligustici Wallichii (*Chuan Xiong*), Radix Rubrus Paeoniae Lactiflorae (*Chi Shao*), Semen Pruni Persicae (*Tao Ren*), and Flos Carthami Tinctorii (*Hong Hua*) as in *Tao Hong Si Wu Tang* (Persica & Carthamus Four Materials Decoction). If there is simultaneous liver depression qi stagnation, Radix Angelicae Sinensis can be combined with Rhizoma Cyperi Rotundi (*Xiang Fu*), Radix Bupleuri (*Chai Hu*), and Tuber Curcumae (*Yu Jin*) as in *Xuan Yu Tong Jing Tang* (Diffuse Depression & Free the Flow of the Channels Decoction).

3. Used for various kinds of static blood aching and pain and for wind damp impediment pain. For the treatment of static blood causing pain in the extremities, Radix Angelicae Sinensis can be combined with Radix Salviae Miltiorrhizae (*Dan Shen*), Resina Olibani (*Ru Xiang*), and Resina Myrrhae (*Mo Yao*) as in *Huo Luo Xiao Ling Dan* (Quicken the Network Vessels Cleverly Effective Elixir). For the treatment of detriment and damage due to fall and strike with stasis, swelling, aching, and pain, Radix Angelicae Sinensis is commonly combined with Radix Et Rhizoma Rhei (*Da Huang*), Semen Pruni Persicae (*Tao Ren*), and Flos Carthami Tinctorii (*Hong Hua*) as in *Fu Yuan Huo Xue Tang* (Restore the Source & Quicken the Blood Decoction). For the treatment of wind damp shoulder and upper arm aching and pain, Radix Angelicae Sinensis is often combined with Radix Et Rhizoma Notopterygii (*Qiang Huo*), Radix Ledebouriellae Divaricatae (*Fang Feng*), and Rhizoma Curcumae Longae (*Jiang Huang*) as in *Juan Bi Tang* (Alleviate Impediment Decoction). For the treatment of numbness of the extremities, Radix Angelicae Sinensis is commonly combined with Caulis Milletiae Seu Spatholobi (*Ji Xue Teng*) and Ramulus Loranthi Seu Visci (*Sang Ji Sheng*).

4. Used for welling and flat abscesses, sores and open sores. For the initial stage or redness, swelling, aching, and pain but no transformation of pus, Radix Angelicae Sinensis should be combined with Flos Lonicerae Japonicae (*Jin Yin Hua*), Radix Rubrus Paeoniae Lactiflorae (*Chi Shao*), and Radix Trichosanthis Kirlowii (*Tian Hua Fen*) as in *Xian Fang Huo Ming Yin* (Immortal Formula Quicken Destiny Drink). During the middle stage when pus is formed but there is not yet eruption, it should be combined with Squama Manitis Pentadactylis (*Chuan Shan Jia*), Spina Gleditschiae Chinensis (*Zao Jiao Ci*), and Radix Astragali Membranacei (*Huang Qi*) as in *Tuo Nong San* (Out-thrust Pus Powder). After rupture, if, due to qi and blood insufficiency, there is not constraining of the mouth for a long time, Radix Angelicae Sinensis should be combined with Radix Astragali Membranacei (*Huang Qi*), Radix Panacis Ginseng (*Ren Shen*), cooked Radix Rehmanniae (*Shu Di*), and Radix Albus Paeoniae Lactiflorae (*Bai Shao*) as in *Shi Quan Da Bu Tang* (Ten [Ingredients] Completely & Greatly Supplementing Decoction).

5. Used for blood vacuity intestinal dryness constipation, Radix Angelicae Sinensis is commonly combined with Herba Cistanchis Deserticolae (*Rou Cong Rong*), uncooked Radix Polygoni Multiflori (*He Shou Wu*), and Semen Cannabis Sativae (*Huo Ma Ren*).

Dosage: 6-15g

Method of use: Decoct in water and administer internally. For supplementing the blood and moistening the intestines, use uncooked. For freeing the flow of the channels and quickening the blood, one can use alcohol stir-fried.

Cautions & contraindications: It is not appropriate to use this medicinal for those with damp exuberance center fullness or loose stools and diarrhea.

Cooked Radix Rehmanniae (*Shu Di*)

Nature & flavor: Sweet and slightly warm

Channel entry: Heart, liver, and kidneys

Functions: Nourishes the blood and enriches yin, supplements the essence and boosts the marrow

Indications:

1. Used for blood vacuity sallow yellow facial complexion, dizziness, heart palpitations, insomnia, menstrual irregularity, and flooding and leaking, cooked Radix Rehmanniae is commonly combined with Radix Angelicae Sinensis (*Dang Gui*), Radix Albus Paeoniae Lactiflorae (*Bai Shao*), and Radix Ligustici Wallichii (*Chuan Xiong*) as in *Si Wu Tang* (Four Materials Decoction).

2. Used for kidney yin insufficiency resulting in tidal heat, night sweats, seminal emission, and wasting and thirsting, cooked Radix Rehmanniae is commonly combined with Radix Dioscoreae Oppositae (*Shan Yao*) and Fructus Corni Officinalis (*Shan Zhu Yu*) as in *Liu Wei Di Huang Wan* (Six Flavors Rehmannia Pills).

3. Used for essence and blood debility and vacuity resulting in dizziness and blurred vision, tinnitus, deafness, and premature whitening of the hair, cooked Radix Rehmanniae is commonly combined with Radix Polygoni Multiflori (*He Shou Wu*), Fructus Ligustri Lucidi (*Nu Zhen Zi*), Herba Ecliptae Prostratae (*Han Lian Cao*), and Fructus Corni Officinalis (*Shan Zhu Yu*).

Dosage: 12-30 g. In large doses, up to 30-60g can be used.

Method of use: Decoct in water and administer internally.

Cautions & contraindications: This ingredient's nature is sticky and slimy and can block dispersion and transformation, *i.e.*, digestion. Therefore, it should not be administered in those with qi stagnation, profuse phlegm, stomach duct and abdominal distention and fullness, scanty eating, or loose stools.

Radix Polygoni Multiflori (*He Shou Wu*)

Nature & flavor: Bitter, sweet, astringent, and slightly warm

Channel entry: Liver and kidneys

Functions: Supplements and boosts the essence and blood, cures malaria, resolves toxins, moistens the intestines and frees the flow of the stool

Indications:

1. Used for essence and blood debility and vacuity dizziness, blurred vision, premature whitening of the hair, low back ache and lower leg flaccidity, and seminal emission and slippery discharge, Radix Polygoni Multiflori is commonly combined with Radix Angelicae Sinensis (*Dang Gui*), Fructus Lycii Chinensis (*Gou Qi Zi*), and Semen Cuscutae Chinensis (*Tu Si Zi*) as in *Qi Bao Mei Ran Dan* (Seven Treasures Beautiful Beard Elixir). For liver-kidney yin vacuity with liver yang tending to be hyperactive and symptoms of dizziness, vertigo, and numbness of the extremities, Radix Polygoni Multiflori can be combined with Fructus Ligustri Lucidi (*Nu Zhen Zi*), Ramulus Loranthi Seu Visci (*Sang Ji Sheng*), Radix Albus Paeoniae Lactiflorae (*Bai Shao*), and Herba Siegesbeckiae (*Xi Xian Cao*).

2. Used for qi and blood dual vacuity enduring malaria which will not stop, Radix Polygoni Multiflori is commonly combined with Radix Panacis Ginseng (*Ren Shen*), Radix Angelicae Sinensis (*Dang Gui*), and Pericarpium Citri Reticulatae (*Chen Pi*) as in *He Ren Yin* (Polygonum & Ginseng Drink).

3. Used for sores and swelling and scrofula. For the former, Radix Polygoni Multiflori can be combined with Radix Sophorae Flavescentis (*Ku Shen*), Herba Menthae Haplocalycis (*Bo He*), and Herba Taraxaci Mongolici Cum Radice (*Pu Gong Ying*). For the latter, it can be combined with Spica Prunellae Vulgaris (*Xia Ku Cao*), Bulbus Fritillariae Thunbergii (*Zhe Bei Mu*), and Radix Scrophulariae Ningpoensis (*Xuan Shen*). For the treatment of scabies, tinea, and itching, Radix Polygoni Multiflori can be combined with Folium Artemisiae Argyii (*Ai Ye*), decocted and used as a wash externally.

4. Used for blood vacuity intestinal dryness constipation, Radix Polygoni Multiflori is commonly combined with Radix Angelicae Sinensis (*Dang Gui*) and Semen Cannabis Sativae (*Huo Ma Ren*).

Dosage: 10-30g

Method of use: For supplementing and boosting the essence and blood, use processed. For curing malaria, resolving toxins, and moistening the intestines, use uncooked. Fresh Radix Polygoni Multiflori is even better for resolving toxins and moistening the intestines.

Cautions & contraindications: It is not appropriate to use this medicinal in those with loose stools and diarrhea or relatively heavy dampness and phlegm.

Radix Albus Paeoniae Lactiflorae (*Bai Shao*)

Nature & flavor: Bitter, sour, and slightly cold

Channel entry: Liver and spleen

Functions: Nourishes the blood and regulates menstruation, constrains yin and stops sweating, emolliates the liver and stops pain, levels and represses liver yang

Indications:

1. Used for blood vacuity menstrual irregularity, painful menstruation, and flooding and leaking, Radix Albus Paeoniae Lactiflorae is commonly combined with Radix Angelicae Sinensis (*Dang Gui*), Radix Ligustici Wallichii (*Chuan Xiong*), and cooked Radix Rehmanniae (*Shu Di*) as in *Si Wu Tang* (Four Materials Decoction).

2. Used for exterior vacuity spontaneous perspirations and yin vacuity night sweats. For the former, Radix Albus Paeoniae Lactiflorae should be combined with Ramulus Cinnamomi Cassiae (*Gui Zhi*). For the latter, it can be combined with Concha Ostreae (*Mu Li*), Os Draconis (*Long Gu*), and Semen Biotae Orientalis (*Bai Zi Ren*).

3. Used for liver qi disharmony with rib-side, flank, stomach duct, and abdominal aching and pain or cramping and pain of the four limbs. For the treatment of liver depression rib-side pain, Radix Albus Paeoniae Lactiflorae is commonly combined with Radix Bupleuri (*Chai Hu*) and Rhizoma Cyperi Rotundi (*Xiang Fu*) as in *Chai Hu Shu Gan Tang* (Bupleurum Course the Liver Decoction). For the treatment of abdominal pain and diarrhea, it can be combined with Rhizoma Atractylodis Macrocephalae (*Bai Zhu*), Pericarpium Citri Reticulatae (*Chen Pi*), and Radix Ledebouriellae Divaricatae (*Fang Feng*) as in *Tong Xie Yao Fang* (Painful Diarrhea Essential Formula). For the treatment of dysentery abdominal pain, Radix Albus Paeoniae Lactiflorae can be combined with Radix Auklandiae Lappae (*Mu Xiang*), Semen Arecae Catechu (*Bing Lang*), and Rhizoma Coptidis Chinensis (*Huang Lian*). For the treatment of stomach duct and abdominal spasm, cramping, aching and pain and cramping and pain of the four extremities, Radix Albus

Paeoniae Lactiflorae is commonly combined with Radix Glycyrrhizae (*Gan Cao*) as in *Shao Yao Gan Cao Tang* (Peony & Licorice Decoction).

4. Used for ascendant liver yang hyperactivity with headache and dizziness, Radix Albus Paeoniae Lactiflorae is commonly combined with uncooked Radix Rehmanniae (*Sheng Di*), Radix Achyranthis Bidentatae (*Niu Xi*), and Haemititum (*Dai Zhe Shi*) as in *Jian Ling Tang* (Fortify the Water Jar Decoction).

Dosage: 6-12g. In larger doses, up to 15-30g can be used.

Method of use: Decoct in water and administer internally. For constraining yin and leveling the liver or treating dysentery, mostly use uncooked. For emolliating the liver and stopping pain, mostly use stir-fried. Stir-frying in alcohol can reduce this medicinal's cold nature.

Cautions & contraindications: This medicinal should not be used alone in case of yang decline vacuity cold conditions. It opposes or reverses Radix Et Rhizoma Veratri (*Li Lu*).

Gelatinum Corii Asini (*E Jiao*)

Nature & flavor: Sweet and level

Channel entry: Lungs, liver, and kidneys

Functions: Supplements the blood and stops bleeding, enriches yin and moistens dryness

Indications:

1. Used for blood vacuity dizziness and heart palpitations, Gelatinum Corii Asini is commonly combined with uncooked Radix Rehmanniae (*Shu Di*), Radix Angelicae Sinensis (*Dang Gui*), Radix Astragali Membranacei (*Huang Qi*), and Radix Codonopsitis Pilosulae (*Dang Shen*) .

2. Used for spitting blood, hacking blood, spontaneous ejection of blood, hemafecia, and flooding and leaking, Gelatinum Corii Asini is especially appropriate for conditions which endure for many days and do not heal with simultaneous yin and blood debility and vacuity. This medicinal can be used alone, dissolved, and taken or it may be combined with other medicinals depending on the disease condition. For the treatment of spitting and hacking of blood, it can be combined with Tuber Ophiopogonis Japonici (*Mai Dong*) and uncooked Radix Rehmanniae (*Sheng Di*). For the treatment of spleen-stomach yang

vacuity hemafecia, it is commonly combined with Rhizoma Atractylodis Macrocephalae (*Bai Zhu*), Radix Lateralis Praeparatus Aconiti Carmichaeli (*Fu Zi*), and Terra Flava Usta (*Fu Long Gan*) as in *Huang Tu Tang* (Yellow Earth Decoction). For the treatment of women's flooding and leaking, excessively profuse menstruation, precipitation of blood during pregnancy, or precipitation of blood after a miscarriage which will not stop, Gelatinum Corii Asini is commonly combined with uncooked Radix Rehmanniae (*Sheng Di*), Radix Albus Paeoniae Lactiflorae (*Bai Shao*), and Folium Artemisiae Argyii (*Ai Ye*) as in *Jiao Ai Tang* (Donkey Skin Glue & Mugwort Decoction).

3. Used for yin vacuity heart vexation and insomnia, Gelatinum Corii Asini is commonly combined with Rhizoma Coptidis Chinensis (*Huang Lian*), Radix Albus Paeoniae Lactiflorae (*Bai Shao*), and chicken egg yolk as in *Huang Lian E Jiao Tang* (Coptis & Donkey Skin Glue Decoction).

4. Used for vacuity taxation panting and coughing or yin vacuity dry cough, Gelatinum Corii Asini is commonly combined with Radix Glehniae Littoralis (*Sha Shen*), Tuber Ophiopogonis Japonici (*Mai Men Dong*), Folium Mori Albi (*Sang Ye*), and Semen Pruni Armeniacae (*Xing Ren*).

Dosage: 6-15g

Method of use: Melted and mixed into the decoction, dissolved in boiling water and taken, or dissolved in yellow wine and taken. For supplementing the blood and enriching yin, it is ok to use this medicinal uncooked. For stopping bleeding, it should be stir-fried in Pollen Typhae (*Pu Huang*). For moistening the lungs, it should be stir-fried in clam shell powder.

Cautions & contraindications: This ingredient's nature is sticky and slimy and can block dispersion and transformation. Therefore, this medicinal is not appropriate for administration to those with spleen-stomach vacuity weakness with no thought for food or drink or vomiting and diarrhea.

Arillus Euphoriae Longanae (*Long Yan Rou*)

Nature & flavor: Sweet and warm

Channel entry: Heart and spleen

Functions: Supplements and boosts the heart and spleen, nourishes the blood and quiets the spirit

Indications: Used for qi and blood insufficiency heart palpitations, racing heart, impaired memory, insomnia, and sallow yellow facial complexion, Arillus Euphoriae

Longanae is commonly combined with Radix Astragali Membranacei (*Huang Qi*), Radix Codonopsitis Pilosulae (*Dang Shen*), and Radix Angelicae Sinensis (*Dang Gui*) as in *Gui Pi Tang* (Return the Spleen Decoction).

Dosage: 10-15g

Method of use: Decoct in water and administer internally.

D. Yin-supplementing medicinals

Radix Glehniae Littoralis (*Sha Shen*)

Nature & flavor: Sweet, slightly bitter, and slightly cold

Channel entry: Lungs and stomach

Functions: Clears the lungs and nourishes yin, boosts the stomach and engenders fluids

Indications:

1. Used for lung heat and dryness cough or taxation cough hacking of blood. For the former, Radix Glehniae Littoralis is commonly combined with Tuber Ophiopogonis Japonici (*Mai Men Dong*), Rhizoma Polygonati Odorati (*Yu Zhu*), and Folium Mori Albi (*Sang Ye*) as in *Sha Shen Mai Dong Tang* (Glehnia & Ophiopogon Decoction). For the latter, Radix Glehniae Littoralis is often combined with Rhizoma Anemarrhenae Aspheloidis (*Zhi Mu*), Bulbus Fritillariae (*Bei Mu*), Tuber Ophiopogonis Japonici (*Mai Men Dong*), and Carapax Amydae Sinensis (*Bie Jia*).

2. Used for heat disease damaging fluids with dry tongue and oral thirst and devitalized eating and drinking, Radix Glehniae Littoralis is commonly combined with uncooked Radix Rehmanniae (*Sheng Di*) and Tuber Ophiopogonis Japonici (*Mai Men Dong*) as in *Yi Wei Tang* (Boost the Stomach Decoction). If fluid damage is heavier, Radix Glehniae Littoralis can be combined with fresh uncooked Radix Rehmanniae (*Sheng Di*) and fresh Herba Dendrobii (*Shi Hu*).

Dosage: 10-15g

Method of use: Decoct in water and administer internally.

Cautions & contraindications: This medicinal is contraindicated in vacuity cold conditions. It opposes or reverses Radix Et Rhizoma Veratri (*Li Lu*).

Tuber Ophiopogonis Japonici (*Mai Men Dong*)

Nature & flavor: Sweet, slightly bitter, and slightly cold

Channel entry: Lungs, heart, and stomach

Functions: Moistens the lungs and nourishes yin, boosts the stomach and engenders fluids, clears the heart and eliminates vexation, moistens the intestines and frees the flow of the stool

Indications:

1. Used for dry cough with sticky phlegm or taxation cough hacking of blood. For the former, Tuber Ophiopogonis Japonici is commonly combined with Folium Mori Albi (*Sang Ye*), Semen Pruni Armeniacae (*Xing Ren*), Gelatinum Corii Asini (*E Jiao*), and uncooked Gypsum Fibrosum (*Shi Gao*) as in *Qing Zao Jiu Fei Tang* (Clear Dryness & Rescue the Lungs Decoction). For the latter, Tuber Ophiopogonis Japonici is commonly combined with Tuber Asparagi Cochinensis (*Tian Men Dong*) as in *Er Dong Gao* (Two Dongs Paste).

2. Used for stomach yin insufficiency dry tongue and oral thirst, Tuber Ophiopogonis Japonici is commonly combined with Radix Glehniae Littoralis (*Sha Shen*), uncooked Radix Rehmanniae (*Sheng Di*), and Rhizoma Polygonati Odorati (*Yu Zhu*) as in *Yi Wei Tang* (Boost the Stomach Decoction).

3. Used for heart vexation and insomnia. If categorized as heat entering the heart constructive, Tuber Ophiopogonis Japonici is commonly combined with Rhizoma Coptidis Chinensis (*Huang Lian*), Radix Salviae Miltiorrhizae (*Dan Shen*), and Folium Bambusae (*Zhu Ye*) as in *Qing Gong Tang* (Clear the Palace Decoction). If categorized as yin vacuity internal heat, Tuber Ophiopogonis Japonici is commonly combined with Radix Scrophulariae Ningpoensis (*Xuan Shen*), uncooked Radix Rehmanniae (*Sheng Di*), and Semen Zizyphi Spinosae (*Suan Zao Ren*) as in *Tian Wang Bu Xin Dan* (Heavenly Emperor Supplement the Heart Elixir).

4. Used for intestinal dryness constipation, Tuber Ophiopogonis Japonici is commonly combined with uncooked Radix Rehmanniae (*Sheng Di*) and Radix Scrophulariae Ningpoensis (*Xuan Shen*) as in *Zheng Ye Tang* (Increase Humors Decoction).

Dosage: 10-15g

Method of use: Decoct in water and administer internally.

Cautions & contraindications: This medicinal is not appropriate for use in external contraction wind cold or damp phlegm obstructing the lungs cough or for spleen-stomach vacuity cold diarrhea.

Herba Dendrobii (*Shi Hu*)

Nature & flavor: Sweet and slightly cold

Channel entry: Stomach and kidneys

Functions: Nourishes the stomach and engenders fluids, enriches yin and eliminates heat

Indications:

1. Used for heat disease damaging fluids or stomach yin insufficiency resulting in oral dryness and vexatious thirst with a dry, crimson tongue, Herba Dendrobii is commonly combined with Radix Glehniae Littoralis (*Sha Shen*), Tuber Ophiopogonis Japonici (*Mai Dong*), and Rhizoma Polygonati Odorati (*Yu Zhu*). This medicinal can also be used fresh with fresh uncooked Radix Rehmanniae (*Sheng Di*), Tuber Ophiopogonis Japonici (*Mai Men Dong*), and Rhizoma Polygonati Odorati (*Yu Zhu*). Or it can be used fresh with fresh uncooked Radix Rehmanniae (*Sheng Di*), Tuber Ophiopogonis Japonici (*Mai Men Dong*), and Radix Trichosanthis Kirlowii (*Tian Hua Fen*).

2. Used for yin vacuity fluid debility with vacuity heat not receding, Herba Dendrobii can be combined with uncooked Radix Rehmanniae (*Sheng Di*), Radix Cynanchi Baiwei (*Bai Wei*), Tuber Ophiopogonis Japonici (*Mai Men Dong*), and Radix Scrophulariae Ningpoensis (*Xuan Shen*).

In addition, Herba Dendrobii also has the actions of brightening the eyes and strengthening the low back and knees. When combined with Flos Chrysanthemi Morifolii (*Ju Hua*) and Fructus Lycii Chinensis (*Gou Qi Zi*), Herba Dendrobii can be used to treat decreased visual acuity. When combined with cooked Radix Rehmanniae (*Shu Di*) and Radix Achyranthis Bidentatae (*Niu Xi*), it can treat low back and knee flaccidity weakness.

Dosage: 6-15g. When used fresh, 15-30g.

Method of use: When entered into decocted prescriptions, this medicinal should be decocted first. Especially for yin vacuity with a dry tongue, it should be decocted for long time.

Cautions & contraindications: This medicinal can constrain evils and assist dampness. Therefore, it should not be used too early for warm heat disease which has not yet transformed dryness nor for damp warm or damp heat conditions.

Bulbus Lilii (*Bai He*)

Nature & flavor: Sweet and slightly cold

Channel entry: Heart and lungs

Functions: Moistens the lungs and stops cough, clears the heart and quiets the spirit

Indications:

1. Used for lung dryness cough and taxation cough hacking of blood, Bulbus Lilii is commonly combined with uncooked Radix Rehmanniae (*Sheng Di*), Radix Scrophulariae Ningpoensis (*Xuan Shen*), and Bulbus Fritillariae (*Bei Mu*) as in *Bai He Gu Jin Tang* (Lily Secure Metal Decoction).

2. Used for the latter stage of heat disease when remaining heat has not been cleared and there is vacuity vexation, fright palpitations, spirit will abstraction, insomnia, and profuse dreams, Bulbus Lilii is commonly combined with Rhizoma Anemarrhenae Aspheloidis (*Zhi Mu*) or uncooked Radix Rehmanniae (*Sheng Di*) as in *Bai He Zhi Mu Tang* (Lily & Anemarrhena Decoction) or *Bai He Di Huang Tang* (Lily & Rehmannia Decoction).

Dosage: 10-30g

Method of administration: Decoct in water and administer internally. For clearing heat, one should use uncooked. For moistening the lungs, one should use mix-fried.

Cautions & contraindications: This medicinal should not be used for wind cold cough or center cold diarrhea.

Fructus Lycii Chinensis (*Gou Qi Zi*)

Nature & flavor: Sweet and level

Channel entry: Liver, kidneys, and lungs

Functions: Supplements the kidneys and boosts the essence, nourishes the liver and brightens the eyes, enriches yin and moistens the lungs

Indications:

1. Used for kidney vacuity essence debility low back and knee aching and flaccidity and seminal emission, Fructus Lycii Chinensis is commonly combined with Rhizoma Polygonati (*Huang Jing*).

2. Used for liver-kidney yin vacuity dizziness, vertigo, and blurred vision, Fructus Lycii Chinensis is commonly combined with Flos Chrysanthemi Morifolii (*Ju Hua*), cooked Radix Rehmanniae (*Shu Di*), Fructus Corni Officinalis (*Shan Zhu Yu*), and Radix Dioscoreae Oppositae (*Shan Yao*) as in *Qi Ju Di Huang Wan* (Lycium & Chrysanthemum Rehmannia Pills).

3. Used for yin vacuity taxation cough, Fructus Lycii Chinensis can be combined with Bulbus Lilii (*Bai He*), Rhizoma Anemarrhenae Aspheloidis (*Zhi Mu*), and Bulbus Fritillariae (*Bei Mu*).

In addition, this ingredient can be used alone for the treatment of wasting and thirsting when steam-cooked, chewed, and swallowed.

Dosage: 5-15g

Method of use: Decoct in water and administer internally.

Cautions & contraindications: This medicinal is not appropriate for use in spleen vacuity loose stools.

Carapax Amydae Sinensis (*Bie Jia*)

Nature & flavor: Salty and cold

Channel entry: Liver and spleen

Functions: Enriches yin and subdues yang, softens the hard and scatters nodulations

Indications:

1. Used for heat disease damaging yin with vacuity wind internally stirring and symptoms of dizziness, vertigo, and spasms and contractions of the hands and feet, Carapax Amydae Sinensis is commonly combined with Concha Ostreae (*Mu Li*), uncooked Radix Rehmanniae (*Sheng Di*), Gelatinum Corii Asini (*E Jiao*), and Radix Albus Paeoniae

Lactiflorae (*Bai Shao*) as in *Er Jia Fu Mai Tang* (Two Shells Restore the Pulse Decoction).

2. Used for yin vacuity fever, bone-steaming, and night sweats, Carapax Amydae Sinensis is commonly combined with Radix Gentianae Macrophyllae (*Qin Jiao*), Cortex Radicis Lycii Chinensis (*Di Gu Pi*), and Rhizoma Anemarrhenae Aspheloidis (*Zhi Mu)* as in *Qin Jiao Bie Jia San* (Gentiana Macrophylla & Carapax Amydae Powder). For the latter stage of heat disease with yin fluid consumptions and damage and symptoms of night-time heat and morning cool, bodily emaciation, a rapid pulse, and a red tongue with scanty fur, Carapax Amydae Sinensis is commonly combined with Herbae Artemisiae Apiaceae (*Qing Hao*), Cortex Radicis Moutan (*Dan Pi*), and uncooked Radix Rehmanniae (*Sheng Di*) as in *Qing Hao Bie Jia Tang* (Artemisia Apiacea & Carapax Amydae Decoction).

3. Used for hypochondral concretions and lumps, static lumps within the abdomen, and blood stasis blocked menstruation, Carapax Amydae Sinensis is commonly combined with Rhizoma Cyperi Rotundi (*Xiang Fu*), Pericarpium Citri Reticulatae Viride (*Qing Pi*), Rhizoma Sparganii (*San Leng*), and Rhizoma Curcumae Zedoariae (*E Zhu*) as in *Bie Jia Wan* (Carapax Amydae Pills).

Dosage: 10-30g

Method of use: Crush and decoct first. For enriching yin and subduing yang, one should use uncooked. For softening the hard and scattering nodulations, one should use vinegar mix-fried.

Cautions & contraindications: Carapax Amydae Sinensis is contraindicated in case of spleen-stomach yang vacuity with scanty eating and loose stools.

Plastrum Testudinis (*Gui Ban*)

Nature & flavor: Sweet, salty, and cold

Channel entry: Liver, kidneys, and heart

Functions: Enriches yin and subdues yang, boosts the kidneys and fortifies the bones, nourishes the blood and supplements the heart, secures the menses and stops bleeding

Indications:

1. Used for yin vacuity yang hyperactivity dizziness and vertigo or yin vacuity stirring of wind spasms and contractions of the hands and feet. For the former, Plastrum Testudinis is commonly combined with Radix Albus Paeoniae Lactiflorae (*Bai Shao*), Radix

Achyranthis Bidentatae (*Niu Xi*), Os Draconis (*Long Gu*), and Haemititum (*Dai Zhe Shi*) as in *Zhen Gan Xi Feng Tang* (Settle the Liver & Extinguish Wind Decoction). For the latter, Plastrum Testudinis is commonly combined with uncooked Radix Rehmanniae (*Sheng Di*), Tuber Ophiopogonis Japonici (*Mai Men Dong*), Carapax Amydae Sinensis (*Bie Jia*), and Gelatinum Corii Asini (*E Jiao*) as in *Da Ding Feng Zhu* (Greatly Stabilizing Wind Pearls).

2. Used for yin vacuity fire effulgence with symptoms of bone-steaming, tidal heat, night sweats, and seminal emission, Plastrum Testudinis is commonly combined with cooked Radix Rehmanniae (*Shu Di*), Rhizoma Anemarrhenae Aspheloidis (*Zhi Mu*), and Cortex Phellodendri (*Huang Bai*) as in *Da Bu Yin Wan* (Greatly Supplementing Yin Pills).

3. Used for liver-kidney insufficiency not fortifying the sinews and bones with low back and lower leg aching and flaccidity as well as children's non-closure of the fontanels, Plastrum Testudinis is commonly combined with cooked Radix Rehmanniae (*Shu Di*), Os Tigridis (*Hu Gu*), and Radix Albus Paeoniae Lactiflorae (*Bai Shao*) as in *Hu Qian Wan* (Tiger Crouching Pills).

4. Used for heat vacuity fright palpitations, insomnia, and impaired memory, Plastrum Testudinis can be combined with Os Draconis (*Long Gu*), Radix Polygalae Tenuifoliae (*Yuan Zhi*), and Rhizoma Acori Graminei (*Shi Chang Pu*) as in *Kong Sheng Zhen Zhong Dan* (Confucian Sage On the Pillow Elixir).

5. Used for yin vacuity blood heat resulting in flooding and leaking or excessively profuse menstruation, Plastrum Testudinis is commonly combined with Radix Albus Paeoniae Lactiflorae (*Bai Shao*), Cortex Phellodendri (*Huang Bai*), and Rhizoma Cyperi Rotundi (*Xiang Fu*) as in *Gu Jing Wan* (Secure the Menses Pills).

Dosage: 10-30g

Method of use: Crush and decoct first. For enriching yin and administering in decoction, use uncooked. When administering in pills and powders, use mix-fried.

Cautions & contraindications: This medicinal should not be used for spleen-stomach yang vacuity or when external contraction of evil qi has not been resolved. It should be used cautiously in pregnant women.

Tuber Asparagi Cochinensis (*Tian Men Dong*)

Nature & flavor: Sweet, slightly bitter, and cold

Channel entry: Lungs and kidneys

Functions: Nourishes yin and moistens dryness, clears the lungs and engenders fluids

Indications:

1. Used for lung dryness dry cough with sticky phlegm, Tuber Asparagi Cochinensis is commonly combined with Tuber Ophiopogonis Japonici (*Mai Men Dong*), Gelatinum Corii Asini (*E Jiao*), and Bulbus Fritillariae Cirrhosae (*Chuan Bei Mu*) as in *Yue Hua Wan* (Moon Luster Pills).

2. Used for dry throat and oral thirst accompanying a damp heat and simultaneous yin vacuity condition, Tuber Asparagai Cochinensis can be combined with Tuber Ophiopogonis Japonici (*Mai Men Dong*), Herba Dendrobii (*Shi Hu*), Radix Scutellariae Baicalensis (*Huang Qin*), and Herba Artemisiae Capillaris (*Yin Chen Hao*) as in *Gan Lu Yin* (Sweet Dew Drink).

Dosage: 6-12g

Method of use: Decoct in water and administer internally.

Rhizoma Polygonati Odorati (*Yu Zhu*)

Nature & flavor: Sweet and slightly cold

Channel entry: Lungs and stomach

Functions: Nourishes yin and moistens dryness, engenders fluids and stops thirst

Indications: Used for lung-stomach yin damage dry heat cough, dry throat, oral thirst, and internal heat wasting and thirsting, Rhizoma Polygonati Odorati can be combined with Radix Glehnia Littoralis (*Sha Shen*) and tuber Ophiopogonis Japonici (*Mai Men Dong*).

Dosage: 6-12g. In large doses, one may use up to 30g.

Method of use: Decoct in water and administer internally.

Herba Ecliptae Prostatae (*Han Lian Cao*)

Nature & flavor: Sweet, sour, and cold

Channel entry: Liver and kidneys

Functions: Enriches and supplements the liver and kidneys, cools the blood and stops bleeding

Indications:

1. Used for liver-kidney yin vacuity with dizziness, blurred vision, tinnitus, and premature greying of the hair, Herba Ecliptae Prostratae is commonly combined with Fructus Ligustri Lucidi (*Nu Zhen Zi*) as in *Er Zhi Wan* (Two Ultimates Pills).

2. Used for yin vacuity blood heat spitting of blood, spontaneous ejection of blood, hematuria, bloody dysentery, and flooding and leaking downward of the blood. For the treatment of hematuria, Herba Ecliptae Prostratae can be combined with Semen Plantaginis (*Che Qian Zi*) and Semen Abutiloni Seu Malvae (*Dong Kui Zi*). For the treatment of hemafecia, Herba Ecliptae Prostratae can be combined with Radix Sanguisorbae (*Di Yu*). For the treatment of women's flooding and leaking or hacking of blood, Herba Ecliptae can be combined with Gelatinum Corii Asini (*E Jiao*) and uncooked Radix Rehmanniae (*Sheng Di*). And for the treatment of spitting of blood, this medicinal can be combined with Cacumen Biotae Orientalis (*Ce Bai Ye*).

In addition, for external bleeding, the fresh herb may be mashed and applied externally.

Dosage: 6-12g. Externally, use a suitable amount.

Method of use: Decoct in water and administer internally.

Fructus Ligustri Lucidi (*Nu Zhen Zi*)

Nature & flavor: Sweet, bitter, and cool

Channel entry: Liver and kidneys

Functions: Enriches and supplements the liver and kidneys, brightens the eyes and blackens the hair

Indications:

1. Used for liver-kidney yin vacuity with dizziness, blurred vision, tinnitus, and premature greying of the hair, Fructus Ligustri Lucidi is commonly combined with Herba Ecliptae

Prostratae (*Han Lian Cao*) as in *Er Zhi Wan* (Two Ultimates Pills).

2. Used for low back and knee soreness and flaccidity, Fructus Ligustri Lucidi can be combined with Fructus Psoraleae Corylifoliae (*Bu Gu Zhi*) and Semen Cuscutae Chinensis (*Tu Si Zi*).

Dosage: 6-12g

Method of administration: Decoct in water and administer internally.

Restraining & astringing medicinals

Medicinals whose main action is to restrain, constrain, secure, and astringe are called restraining and astringing medicinals. The medicinals in this category are mostly sour-flavored or astringent-flavored. They are divided into those which secure the exterior and constrain sweating, those which astringe the intestines and stop diarrhea, those which secure the essence and reduce urination, those which constrain the lungs and stop coughing, and those which stop bleeding and stop abnormal vaginal discharge. Such medicinals are suitable for use in enduring disease bodily vacuity and insecurity of the righteous qi resulting in such conditions of slippery desertion and lack of prohibition as spontaneous perspiration, night sweats, enduring diarrhea, seminal emission, slippery essence, urinary incontinence, frequent urination, enduring cough, vacuity panting, and flooding and leaking and abnormal vaginal discharge which will not stop.

Because the root cause of slippery desertion conditions is a righteous qi vacuity weakness, therefore, the medicinals in this class should be combined with other appropriate supplementing and boosting medicinals. For instance, for qi vacuity spontaneous perspiration, restraining and astringing medicinals should be combined with qi-supplementing ingredients. For yin vacuity night sweats, they should be combined with yin-nourishing medicinals. For spleen vacuity enduring diarrhea, they should be combined with spleen-fortifying medicinals. And for kidney vacuity seminal emission, they should be combined with kidney-supplementing medicinals.

Because restraining and astringing medicinals can constrain evils as well as the righteous, they are not appropriate for use in case of replete evils.

Fructus Levis Tritici Aestivi (*Fu Xiao Mai*)

Nature & flavor: Sweet and cool

Channel entry: Heart

Functions: Boosts the qi, eliminates heat, and stops sweating

Indications:

1. Used for spontaneous perspiration and night sweats. When used alone, this ingredient is stir-fried till scorched, ground into powder, and taken frequently. Or it may be combined

with other medicinals. For the treatment of exterior vacuity spontaneous perspiration, Fructus Levis Tritici Aestivi can be combined with Radix Astragali Membranacei (*Huang Qi*) and Fructus Schisandrae Chinensis (*Wu Wei Zi*). For the treatment of yin vacuity night sweats, it can be combined with Radix Albus Paeoniae Lactiflorae (*Bai Shao*) and Fructus Corni Officinalis (*Shan Zhu Yu*).

2. Used for bone-steaming and taxation heat, Fructus Levis Tritici Aestivi can be combined with uncooked Radix Rehmanniae (*Sheng Di*), Tuber Ophiopogonis Japonici (*Mai Men Dong*), and Cortex Radicis Lycii Chinensis (*Di Gu Pi*).

Dosage: 15-30g. When stir-fried till scorched, ground, and taken, take 3-6g each time.

Method of use: Decoct in water and administer internally.

Cautions & contraindications: This medicinal should not be used if there are exterior evils.

Fructus Schisandrae Chinensis (*Wu Wei Zi*)

Nature & flavor: Sour, sweet, and warm

Channel entry: Lungs, heart, and kidneys

Functions: Constrains the lungs and enriches the kidneys, engenders fluids and constrains the sweat, astringes the essence and stops diarrhea, calms the heart and quiets the spirit

Indications:

1. Used for enduring cough and vacuity panting. For the former, Fructus Schisandrae Chinensis is often combined with Pericarpium Papaveris (*Ying Su Ke*) and Fructus Pruni Mume (*Wu Mei*). For the latter, Fructus Schisandrae Chinensis is commonly combined with cooked Radix Rehmanniae (*Shu Di*), Fructus Corni Officinalis (*Shan Zhu Yu*), and Radix Dioscoreae Oppositae (*Shan Yao*) as in *Du Qi Wan* (All Qi Pills).

2. Used for fluid damage oral thirst, spontaneous perspiration, and night sweats. For the treatment of heat damaging the qi and yin, Fructus Schisandrae Chinensis is commonly combined with Radix Panacis Ginseng (*Ren Shen*) and Tuber Ophiopogonis Japonici (*Mai Men Dong*) as in *Sheng Mai San* (Engender the Pulse Powder). For the treatment of vacuity sweating which will not stop, Fructus Schisandrae Chinensis is commonly combined with Semen Biotae Orientalis (*Bai Zi Ren*), Radix Panacis Ginseng (*Ren Shen*), Radix Ephedrae (*Ma Huang Gen*), and Concha Ostreae (*Mu Li*) as in *Bai Zi Ren Wan*

(Biota Seed Pills). For the treatment of wasting and thirsting condition, it may be combined with Radix Astragali Membranacei (*Huang Qi*), uncooked Radix Rehmanniae (*Sheng Di*), Tuber Ophiopogonis Japonici (*Mai Dong*), and Radix Trichosanthis Kirlowii (*Tian Hua Fen*) as in *Huang Qi Tang* (Astragalus Decoction).

3. Used for seminal emission and slippery essence, Fructus Schisandrae Chinensis can be used alone or it may be combined with Ootheca Mantidis (*Sang Piao Xiao*) and Os Draconis (*Long Gu*) as in *Sang Piao Xiao Wan* (Mantis Eggcase Pills).

4. Used for spleen-kidney vacuity cold fifth watch diarrhea, Fructus Schisandrae is commonly combined with Fructus Psoraleae Corylifoliae (*Bu Gu Zhi*), Fructus Evodiae Rutecarpae (*Wu Zhu Yu*), and Semen Myristicae Fragrantis (*Rou Dou Kou*) as in *Si Shen Wan* (Four Spirits Pills).

5. Used for heart blood insufficiency and kidney yin debility and vacuity resulting in vacuity vexation, heart palpitations, insomnia, and profuse dreams, Fructus Schisandrae Chinensis is commonly combined with uncooked Radix Rehmanniae (*Shu Di*), Tuber Ophiopogonis Japonici (*Mai Dong*), Radix Salviae Miltiorrhizae (*Dan Shen*), and Semen Zizyphi Spinosae (*Suan Zao Ren*) as in *Tian Wang Bu Xin Dan* (Heavenly Emperor Supplement the Heart Elixir).

In addition, when this ingredient is ground into powder and taken internally for the treatment of chronic hepatitis with high GPT levels, its effect is to lower the GPT.

Dosage: 3-10g. Use 1.5-3g for constraining the lungs and settling cough, while for enriching, supplementing, and boosting yin, use 6-10g.

Method of use: Decoct in water and administer internally. Take 1-3g each time when ground into powder.

Cautions & contraindications: Because this ingredient is sour, astringent, restraining, and constraining, it should not be used in those with exterior evils which have not been resolved, for those with internal replete heat, for the initial stage of cough, nor for the initial emission of measles rash.

Fructus Pruni Mume (*Wu Mei*)

Nature & flavor: Sour, astringent, and level

Channel entry: Liver, spleen, lungs, and large intestine

Functions: Constrains the lungs and stops cough, astringes the intestines and stops diarrhea, engenders fluids and stops thirst, harmonizes the stomach and quiets roundworms

Indications:

1. Used for lung vacuity enduring cough, Fructus Pruni Mume is commonly combined with Pericarpium Papaveris Somniferi (*Ying Su Ke*), Rhizoma Pinelliae Ternatae (*Ban Xia*), Semen Pruni Armeniacae (*Xing Ren*), and Gelatinum Corii Asini (*E Jiao*) as in *Yi Fu San* (One Administration Powder).

2. Used for enduring diarrhea and enduring dysentery, Fructus Pruni Mume is commonly combined with Semen Myristicae Fragrantis (*Rou Dou Kou*), Radix Codonopsitis Pilosulae (*Dang Shen*), and Fructus Terminaliae Chebulae (*He Zi*) as in *Gu Chang Wan* (Secure the Intestines Pills).

3. Used for vacuity heat wasting and thirsting, Fructus Pruni Mume is commonly combined with Radix Trichosanthis Kirlowii (*Tian Hua Fen*), Tuber Ophiopogonis Japonici (*Mai Men Dong*), Radix Puerariae (*Ge Gen*), and Radix Panacis Ginseng (*Ren Shen*) in *Yu Quan Wan* (Jade Spring Pills).

4. Used for intestinal roundworms leading to the arising of abdominal pain and vomiting, Fructus Pruni Mume is commonly combined with Herba Asari Cum Radice (*Xi Xin*), Fructus Zanthoxyli Bungeani (*Hua Jiao*), dry Rhizoma Zingiberis (*Gan Jiang*), and Rhizoma Coptidis Chinensis (*Huang Lian*) as in *Wu Mei Wan* (Mume Pills). For biliary ascariasis, it may be combined with Herba Artemisiae Capillaris (*Yin Chen Hao*).

In addition, this ingredient also has an action of stopping bleeding and can be used in the treatment of hemafecia, hematuria, and flooding and leaking precipitation of blood. Externally applied, it is able to disperse sore swelling and treats ophthalmic pterygium.

Dosage: 3-10g. In large doses, it can be used up to 30g. Externally, use a suitable amount.

Method of use: Decoct in water and administer internally. For stopping bleeding and stopping diarrhea, it should be stir-fried till carbonized. For engendering fluids and quieting roundworms, use uncooked.

Cautions & contraindications: Because this ingredient's sour, constraining nature is relatively strong, it is not appropriate for use if externally there are exterior evils or internally is there is replete heat, accumulation, and stagnation.

Semen Nelumbinis Nuciferae (*Lian Zi*)

Nature & flavor: Sweet, astringent, and level

Channel entry: Spleen, kidneys, and heart

Functions: Supplements the spleen and stops diarrhea, boosts the kidneys and secures the essence, nourishes the heart and quiets the spirit

Indications:

1. Used for spleen vacuity enduring diarrhea and devitalized eating and drinking, Semen Nelumbinis Nuciferae is commonly combined with Radix Panacis Ginseng (*Ren Shen*), Rhizoma Atractylodis Macrocephalae (*Bai Zhu*), Sclerotium Poriae Cocos (*Fu Ling*), and Radix Dioscoreae Oppositae (*Shan Yao*) as in *Shen Ling Bai Zhu San* (Ginseng, Poria & Atractylodes Powder).

2. Used for kidney vacuity seminal emission and slippery essence, Semen Nelumbinis Nuciferae is commonly combined with Semen Astragali Complanati (*Sha Yuan Zi*), Os Draconis (*Long Gu*), and Concha Ostreae (*Mu Li*) as in *Jin Suo Gu Jing Wan* (Golden Lock Secure the Essence Pills).

3. Used for vacuity vexation, fright palpitations, and insomnia, Semen Nelumbinis Nuciferae can be combined with Semen Zizyphi Spinosae (*Suan Zao Ren*), Radix Polygalae Tenuifoliae (*Yuan Zhi*), and Sclerotium Poriae Cocos (*Fu Ling*).

In addition, this medicinal can be used for women's flooding and leaking and excessively profuse vaginal discharge conditions.

Dosage: 6-15g

Method of use: Decoct in water and administer internally.

Cautions & contraindications: This medicinal should not be used if there is large intestine dryness and binding.

Fructus Corni Officinalis (*Shan Zhu Yu*)

Nature & flavor: Sour and slightly warm

Channel entry: Liver and kidneys

Functions: Supplements and boosts the liver and kidneys, restrains, constrains, secures, and astringes

Indications:

1. Used for liver-kidney debility and vacuity dizziness and vertigo, low back and knee aching and flaccidity, impotence, seminal emission, frequent urination, and urinary incontinence. If categorized as liver-kidney yin debility, Fructus Corni Officinalis is commonly combined with cooked Radix Rehmanniae (*Shu Di*) and Radix Dioscoreae Oppositae (*Shan Yao*) as in *Liu Wei Di Huang Wan* (Six Flavors Rehmannia Pills). If categorized as kidney yang insufficiency, it can be combined with Fructus Psoraleae Corylifoliae (*Bu Gu Zhi*) and Radix Angelicae Sinensis (*Dang Gui*) as in *Cao Huan Dan* (Herbal Restorative Elixir). For the treatment of urinary incontinence, Fructus Corni Officinalis can be combined with Ootheca Mantidis (*Sang Piao Xiao*), Fructus Rubi Chingii (*Fu Pen Zi*), Fructus Alpiniae Oxyphyllae (*Yi Zhi Ren*), and Semen Astragali Complanati (*Sha Yuan Zi*).

2. Used for great sweating which will not stop and bodily vacuity on the verge of desertion, Fructus Corni Officinalis is commonly combined with Radix Panacis Ginseng (*Ren Shen*), Radix Lateralis Praeparatus Aconiti Carmichaeli (*Fu Zi*), Os Draconis (*Long Gu*), and Concha Ostreae (*Mu Li*).

3. Used for women's flooding and leaking and excessively profuse menstruation, Fructus Corni Officinalis can be combined with Os Sepiae Seu Sepiellae (*Wu Zei Gu*), carbonized Radix Rubiae Cordifoliae (*Qian Cao*), and carbonized Stipulae Trachycarpi (*Zong Lu*) as in *Gu Chong Tang* (Secure the *Chong* Decoction).

Dosage: 5-10g. In large doses, this medicinal can be used up to 30g.

Method of use: Decoct in water and administer internally.

Cautions & contraindications: This ingredient is warming, supplementing, restraining, and constraining. Therefore, it should not be used for liver yang tending towards hyperactivity, if there is habitual damp heat, or for inhibited urination.

Fructus Alpiniae Oxyphyllae (*Yi Zhi Ren*)

Nature & flavor: Acrid and warm

Channel entry: Spleen and kidneys

Functions: Warms the spleen, opens the stomach, and contains drool, warms the kidneys, secures the essence, and reduces urination

Indications:

1. Used for spleen-stomach yang vacuity abdominal pain, vomiting, and diarrhea, scanty eating, and profuse sleeping, Fructus Alpiniae Oxyphyllae can be combined with Radix Codonopsitis Pilosulae (*Dang Shen*), Rhizoma Atractylodis Macrocephalae (*Bai Zhu*), dry Rhizoma Zingiberis (*Gan Jiang*), and Pericarpium Citri Reticulatae (*Chen Pi*).

2. Used for kidney qi vacuity cold seminal emission, urinary incontinence, terminal dribbling or urination, and increased night-time urination, Fructus Alpiniae Oxyphyllae is commonly combined with Radix Dioscoreae Oppositae (*Shan Yao*) and Radix Linderae Strychnifoliae (*Wu Yao*) as in *Suo Quan Wan* (Reduce the Spring Pills)

Dosage: 3-6g

Method of use: Decoct in water and administer internally.

Cautions & contraindications: This ingredient is drying and hot and easily damages yin and invigorates fire. Therefore, it is contraindicated in yin vacuity fire effulgence and conditions categorized as damp heat.

Os Sepiae Seu Sepiellae (*Wu Zei Gu*)

Nature & flavor: Salty, astringent, and slightly warm

Channel entry: Liver, kidneys, and stomach

Functions: Restrains, constrains, and stops bleeding, secures the essence and stop vaginal discharge, controls acidity and stops pain, restrains dampness and constrains sores

Indications:

1. Used for flooding and leaking precipitation of blood and bleeding due to injury by metal, *i.e.*, cuts. For the former, Os Sepiae Seu Sepiellae is commonly combined with

Radix Rubiae Cordifoliae (*Qian Cao*), carbonized Petiolus Trachycarpi (*Zong Lu*), and Galla Rhois Chinensis (*Wu Bei Zi*) as in *Gu Chong Tang* (Secure the *Chong* Decoction). For the latter, Os Sepiae Seu Sepiellae can be used alone when ground into powder and applied externally.

2. Used for seminal emission and abnormal vaginal discharge. For the former, Os Sepiae Seu Sepiellae can be combined with Fructus Corni Officinalis (*Shan Zhu Yu*), Semen Cuscutae Chinensis (*Tu Si Zi*), and Semen Astragali Complanati (*Sha Yuan Zi*). For the latter, it can be combined with Radix Angelicae Dahuricae (*Bai Zhi*) and Crinis Carbonisatus (*Xue Yu Tan*).

3. Used for stomach pain and acid eructations, Os Sepiae Seu Sepiellae is commonly combined with Bulbus Fritillariae Thunbergii (*Zhe Bei Mu*). This is then called *Wei Bei San* (Cuttlefish Bone & Fritillaria Powder). If there is accompanying stomach bleeding, Os Sepiae Seu Sepiellae can be combined with Rhizoma Bletillae Striatae (*Bai Ji*) as in *Wu Ji San* (Cuttlefish Bone & Bletilla Powder).

4. Used for damp sores, eczema, and ulcerated sores with profuse pus, Os Sepiae Seu Sepiellae can be used alone ground into powder and applied externally, or it can be combined with calcined Gypsum Fibrosum (*Shi Gao*), Alum (*Ku Fan*), and Pulvis Indigonis (*Qing Dai*) or Sanguis Draconis (*Xue Jie*).

Dosage: 6-12g. One point five to 3g each time when ground into powder and swallowed. Externally, use a suitable amount.

Method of use: Decoct in water and administer internally or grind into powder and swallow.

Cautions & contraindications: This medicinal should not be used in cases of yin vacuity internal heat and dry, bound stools.

Hallyositum Rubrum (*Chi Shi Zhi*)

Nature & flavor: Sweet, sour, astringent, and warm

Channel entry: Spleen, stomach, and large intestine

Functions: Astringes the intestines, stops bleeding, engenders muscle, *i.e.*, flesh, and constrains, *i.e.*, closes, sores

Indications:

1. Used for enduring diarrhea and enduring dysentery due to vacuity cold, Hallyositum

Rubrum is commonly combined with dry Rhizoma Zingiberis (*Gan Jiang*), Radix Codonopsitis Pilosulae (*Dang Shen*), and Rhizoma Atractylodis Macrocephalae (*Bai Zhu*).

2. Used for women's enduring floodids and leaking due to vacuity cold, Hallyositum Rubrum can be combined with Os Sepiae Seu Sepiellae (*Wu Zei Gu*).

In addition, this medicinal may be powdered and applied externally for the treatment of sores and open sores which will not constrain and eczema with pussy water soaking and pouring, *i.e.*, eczema with exudation.

Dosage: 9-12g. Externally, use a suitable amount.

Method of use: Decoct in water and administer internally or grind into powder and apply externally to the affected area.

Fructus Terminaliae Chebulae (*He Zi*)

Nature & flavor: Bitter, sour, astringent, and level

Channel entry: Lungs, stomach, and large intestine

Functions: Astringes the intestines and constrains the lungs, downbears fire and disinhibits the throat

Indications:

1. Used for spleen-kidney dual vacuity enduring diarrhea and enduring dysentery, Fructus Terminaliae Chebulae can be combined with Rhizoma Atractylodis Macrocephalae (*Bai Zhu*), Semen Euryalis Ferocis (*Qian Shi*), and Semen Myristicae Fragrantis (*Rou Dou Kou*). For the treatment of enduring diarrhea due to vacuity cold, Fructus Terminaliae Chebulae can be combined with dry Rhizoma Zingiberis (*Gan Jiang*) and Pericarpium Papaveris Somniferi (*Ying Su Ke*). For treatment of enduring diarrhea and dysentery due to remaining damp heat evils which have not been cleared, Fructus Terminaliae Chebulae can be combined with Rhizoma Coptidis Chinensis (*Huang Lian*) and Radix Auklandiae Lappae (*Mu Xiang*).

2. Used for bloody stool anal desertion, Fructus Terminaliae Chebulae can be combined with Galla Rhois Chinensis (*Wu Bei Zi*) and Fructus Pruni Mume (*Wu Mei*).

3. Used for lung yin vacuity panting and coughing and enduring, dry cough which will not stop, Fructus Terminaliae Chebulae can be combined with Fructus Schisandrae Chinensis

(*Wu Wei Zi*), Radix Glehniae Littoralis (*Sha Shen*), and Bulbus Lilii (*Bai He*). If there are threads of blood in the phlegm, Fructus Terminaliae Chebulae can be combined with Pumice (*Hai Fu Shi*) and Pericarpium Trichosanthis Kirlowii (*Gua Lou Pi*).

4. Used for enduring sore throat and hoarseness, Fructus Terminaliae Chebulae can be combined with Radix Platycodi Grandiflori (*Jie Geng*) and Radix Glycyrrhizae (*Gan Cao*).

Dosage: 3-10g

Method of use: Decoct in water and administer internally.

Cautions & contraindications: This medicinal is contraindicated in case of external contraction coughing and panting and acute diarrhea and the initial stage of dysentery.

Semen Myristicae Fragrantis (*Rou Dou Kou*)

Nature & flavor: Acrid and warm

Channel entry: Spleen and large intestine

Functions: Warms the center and moves the qi, astringes the intestines and stops diarrhea

Indications:

1. Used for stomach duct and abdominal distention and pain, scanty eating, and vomiting and spitting, Semen Myristicae Fragrantis can be combined with Radix Auklandiae Lappae (*Mu Xiang*).

2. Used for enduring diarrhea and dysentery due to spleen-stomach vacuity cold, Semen Myristicae Fragrantis is commonly combined with Radix Codonopsitis Pilosulae (*Dang Shen*), Rhizoma Atractylodis Macrocephalae (*Bai Zhu*), and dry Rhizoma Zingiberis (*Gan Jiang*). For spleen-kidney dual vacuity fifth watch diarrhea, Semen Myristicae Fragrantis can be combined with Fructus Psoraleae Corylifoliae (*Bu Gu Zhi*).

Dosage: 3-10g

Method of use: Decoct in water and administer internally.

Cautions & contraindication: This medicinal is contraindicated in hot diarrhea and dysentery.

Pericarpium Papaveris Somniferi (*Ying Su Ke*)

Nature & flavor: Sour, astringent, and level. Has toxins.

Channel entry: Lungs, kidneys, and large intestine

Functions: Constrains the lungs, astringes the intestines, and stops pain

Indications:

1. For enduring cough which will not stop, Pericarpium Papaveris Somniferi can be combined with Fructus Pruni Mume (*Wu Mei*) and Fructus Schisandrae Chinensis (*Wu Wei Zi*).

2. For enduring diarrhea and anal desertion with stomach venter and abdominal aching and pain, Pericarpium Papaveris Somniferi can be combined with Rhizoma Coptidis Chinensis (*Huang Lian*) and Radix Auklandiae Lappae (*Mu Xiang*).

Dosage: 3-6g

Method of use: Decoct in water and administer internally. Use uncooked for astringing the intestines and stopping pain. Use stir-fried to constrain the lungs and stop coughing.

Cautions & contraindications: Because this ingredient easily produces addiction, it should not be used regularly, *i.e.*, over an extended period of time.

Semen Euryalis Ferocis (*Qian Shi*)

Nature & flavor: Sweet, astringent, and level

Channel entry: Spleen and kidneys

Functions: Boosts the kidneys and secures the essence, supplements the spleen and stops diarrhea, dispels dampness and stops vaginal discharge

Indications:

1. Used for dream emission and slippery essence, frequent urination and urinary incontinence, Semen Euryalis Ferocis is commonly combined with Fructus Rosae Laevigatae (*Jin Ying Zi*).

2. Used for spleen vacuity enduring diarrhea, white turbidity, and abnormal vaginal discharge, Semen Euryalis Ferocis can be combined with Radix Codonopsitis Pilosulae

(*Dang Shen*), Rhizoma Atractylodis Macrocephalae (*Bai Zhu*), and Sclerotium Poriae Cocos (*Fu Ling*).

3. For the treatment of spleen-kidney dual vacuity vaginal discharge, Semen Eurylais Ferocis can be combined with Radix Dioscoreae Oppositae (*Shan Yao*). For vaginal discharge due to damp heat, it can be combined with Semen Plantaginis (*Che Qian Zi*) and Cortex Phellodendri (*Huang Bai*).

Dosage: 10-15g

Method of use: Decoct in water and administer internally.

Fructus Rosae Laevigatae (*Jin Ying Zi*)

Nature & flavor: Sour, sweet, astringent, and level

Channel entry: Kidneys, urinary bladder, and large intestine

Functions: Secures the essence and reduces urination, astringes the intestines and stops diarrhea

Indications:

1. Used for seminal emission, slippery essence, frequent urination, and urinary incontinence, Fructus Rosae Laevigatae is commonly combined with Semen Euryalis Ferocis (*Qian Shi*). If the above are due to kidney yin vacuity, Fructus Rosae Laevigatae can be combined with Os Draconis (*Long Gu*) and Concha Ostreae (*Mu Li*). This combination can also be used for enduring women's leaking which dribbles and drips without cease.

2. Used for enduring diarrhea and enduring dysentery, Fructus Rosae Laevigatae can be combined with Radix Codonopsitis Pilosulae (*Dang Shen*), Rhizoma Atractylodis Macrocephalae (*Bai Zhu*), and Radix Dioscoreae Oppositae (*Shan Yao*).

Dosage: 6-12g

Method of use: Decoct in water and administer internally.

Fructus Rubi Chingii (*Fu Pen Zi*)

Nature & flavor: Sweet, sour, and warm

Channel entry: Liver and kidneys

Functions: Boosts the kidneys, secures the essence, and reduces urination

Indications:

1. Used for kidney vacuity urinary incontinence and frequent urination, Fructus Rubi Chingii is commonly combined with Ootheca Mantidis (*Sang Piao Xiao*) and Fructus Alpiniae Oxyphyllae (*Yi Zhi Ren*).

2. Used for impotence, premature ejaculation, seminal emission, and slippery essence, Fructus Rubi Chingii can be combined with Semen Cuscutae Chinensis (*Tu Si Zi*), Fructus Schisandrae Chinensis (*Wu Wei Zi*), and Fructus Lycii Chinensis (*Gou Qi Zi*).

Dosage: 6-12g

Method of use: Decoct in water and administer internally.

Galla Rhois Chinensis (*Wu Bei Zi*)

Nature & flavor: Sour, astringent, and cold

Channel entry: Lungs, stomach, and large intestine

Functions: Constrains the lungs and downbears fires, astringes the intestines and stops diarrhea, constrains sweat and stops bleeding, restrains dampness and constrains sores

Indications:

1. Used for lung vacuity enduring cough, Galla Rhois Chinensis is commonly combined with Fructus Schisandrae Chinensis (*Wu Wei Zi*) and Pericarpium Papaveris Somniferi (*Ying Su Ke*).

2. Used for enduring diarrhea and enduring dysentery, Galla Rhois Chinensis can be combined with Fructus Terminaliae Chebulae (*He Zi*) or with Semen Myristicae Fragrantis (*Rou Dou Kou*) and Radix Codonopsitis Pilosulae (*Dang Shen*).

3. Used for night sweats, Galla Rhois Chinensis can be combined with Os Draconis (*Long Gu*) and Concha Ostreae (*Mu Li*).

4. Used for hemafecia and hemorrhoidal bleeding, Galla Rhois Chinensis can be combined with Flos Immaturus Sophorae Japonicae (*Huai Hua Mi*) and Radix Sanguisorbae (*Di Yu*).

5. Used for rectal prolapse due to central qi falling downward, Galla Rhois Chinensis can be combined with Radix Astragali Membranacei (*Huang Qi*), Radix Codonopsitis Pilosulae (*Dang Shen*), Radix Bupleuri (*Chai Hu*), and Rhizoma Cimicifugae (*Sheng Ma*).

In addition, powdered Galla Rhois Chinensis can be used for the treatment of external injury bleeding, welling abscesses, swelling, sores, and toxins when applied externally.

Dosage: 3-6g. Externally, use a suitable amount.

Method of use: Decoct in water and administer internally or powder and apply externally to the affected area.

Semen Ginkgonis Bilobae (*Bai Guo*)

Nature & flavor: Sweet, bitter, astringent, and level. Has toxins.

Channel entry: Lungs and kidneys

Functions: Constrains the lungs and stabilizes panting, stops vaginal discharge and turbidity, reduces urination

Indications:

1. Used for panting and coughing with profuse, yellow phlegm due to lung vacuity with simultaneous hot phlegm, Semen Ginkgonis Bilobae is commonly combined with Herba Ephedrae (*Ma Huang*), Semen Pruni Armeniacae (*Xing Ren*), and Cortex Radicis Mori Albi (*Sang Bai Pi*).

2. Used for damp heat vaginal discharge and white turbidity, Semen Ginkgonis Bilobae can be combined with Cortex Phellodendri (*Huang Bai*) and Semen Euryalis Ferocis (*Qian Shi*).

3. Used for red ans white vaginal discharge and lower source vacuity, Semen Gingkonis Bilobae can be combined with Semen Nelumbinis Nuciferae (*Lian Zi*) and Os Sepiae Seu Sepiellae (*Hai Piao Xiao*).

4. Used for urinary incontinence and frequent urination, Semen Ginkgonis Bilobae can be combined with Ootheca Mantidis (*Sang Piao Xiao*) and Fructus Alpiniae Oxyphyllae (*Yi Zhi Ren*).

Dosage: 4.5-10g

Method of use: Decoct in water and administer internally.

Radix Ephedrae (*Ma Huang Gen*)

Nature & flavor: Sweet and level

Channel entry: Lungs

Functions: Stops sweating

Indications: Used for spontaneous perspiration and night sweats. For the former when due to exterior vacuity, it can be combined with Radix Astragali Membranacei (*Huang Qi*) and Concha Ostreae (*Mu Li*). For the latter when due to yin vacuity, it can be combined with Fructus Schisandrae Chinensis (*Wu Wei Zi*) and Semen Biotae Orientalis (*Bai Zi Ren*).

Dosage: 3-10g

Method of use: Decoct in water and administer internally.

Cautions & contraindications: This medicinal is contraindicate for use in exterior patterns.

Ootheca Mantidis (*Sang Piao Xiao*)

Nature & flavor: Sweet, salty, and level

Channel entry: Liver and kidneys

Functions: Boosts the kidneys and secures the essence, reduces urination, stops turbidity

Indications:

1. Used for seminal emission, slippery essence, urinary incontinence, and frequent urination due to kidney vacuity, Ootheca Mantidis can be combined with Fructus Corni

Officinalis (*Shan Zhu Yu*), Semen Cuscutae Chinensis (*Tu Si Zi*), and Radix Astragali Membranacei (*Huang Qi*). For children's bedwetting, it can be combined with Radix Polygalae Tenuifoliae (*Yuan Zhi*), Radix Codonopsitis Pilosulae (*Dang Shen*), Sclerotium Poriae Cocos (*Fu Ling*), and Radix Angelicae Sinensis (*Dang Gui*).

2. Used for abnormal vaginal discharge, Ootheca Mantidis can be combined with Semen Cuscutae Chinensis (*Tu Si Zi*) and Semen Euryalis Ferocis (*Qian Shi*).

Dosage: 4.5-10g

Method of use: Decoct in water and administer internally; also appropriate for use in pills and powders.

Bibliography

Chinese language bibliography

Ben Cao Tu Jing (The Materia Medica Illustrated Classic), Su Song, Anhui Science & Technology Press, Hefei, 1994

Zhong Yao, Lin Qian-lian, Shanghai Science & Technology Press, Shanghai, 1981

Zhong Yao Cai Se Tu Ji (A Colored Atlas of Chinese Medicinals), ed. by Yao Da-mu & Zhang Jing-bao, Joint Publishing (H.K.) Co., Ltd., Hong Kong, 1996

Zhong Cao Yao Xue (A Study of Chinese Herbs & Medicinals), Shanghai College of Chinese Medicine, Commercial Press, Hong Kong, 1975

Zhong Yao Da Ci Dian (A Great Dictionary of Chinese Medicinals), compiled by the Jiangsu College of New Medicine, Shanghai Science & Technology Press, Shanghai, 1991

Zhong Yao Xue (A Study of Chinese Medicinals), Qu Jing-feng *et al.*, Shanghai College of Chinese Medicine Press, Shanghai, 1994

Zhong Yao Xue (A Study of Chinese Medicinals), Chengdu College of Chinese Medicine, Shanghai Science & Technology Press, Shanghai, 1977

Zhong Yao Xue (A Study of Chinese Medicinals), Gansu Provincial Academy of New Medicine, Peoples Health & Hygiene Press, Beijing, 1982

English language bibliography

A Barefoot Doctor's Manual, Hunan Province Revolutionary Health Committee, Cloudburst Press, Seattle, 1977

A Compendium of TCM Patterns & Treatments, Bob Flaws & Daniel Finney, Blue Poppy Press, Boulder, CO, 1996

Chinese Herbal Medicine: Formulas & Strategies, Dan Bensky & Randall Barolet, Eastland Press, Seattle, 1990

Chinese Herbal Medicine: Materia Medica, Dan Bensky & Andrew Gamble, Eastland Press, Seattle, 1993

Dui Yao: The Art of Combining Chinese Medicinals, Philippe Sionneau, Blue Poppy Press, Boulder, CO, 1997

English-Chinese Chinese-English Dictionary of Chinese Medicine, Nigel Wiseman, Hunan Science & Technology Press, Changsha, 1995

Handbook of Chinese Herbs, Him-che Yeung, self-published, LA, 1996

How to Write a TCM Herbal Formula, Bob Flaws, Blue Poppy Press, Boulder, CO, 1993

Medicine in China: A History of Pharmaceutics, Paul U. Unschuld, Univ. of CA Press, Berkeley, 1986

Oriental Materia Medica: A Concise Guide, Hong-yen Hsu *et al.*, Oriental Healing Arts Institute, Long Beach, CA, 1986

Pao Zhi: An Introduction to the Use of Processed Chinese Medicinals, Blue Poppy Press, Boulder, CO, 1995

Seventy Essential TCM Formulas for Beginners, Bob Flaws, Blue Poppy Press, Boulder, CO, 1994

Statements of Fact in Traditional Chinese Medicine, Bob Flaws, Blue Poppy Press, Boulder, CO, 1994

The Divine Farmer's Materia Medica, Tao Hong-jing, trans. by Yang Shou-zhong, Blue Poppy Press, Boulder, CO 1998

The English-Chinese Encyclopedia of Practical Traditional Chinese Medicine: The Chinese Materia Medica, ed. by Huang Kui-ming *et al.*, Higher Education Press, Beijing, 1994

The Heart Transmission of Medicine, Liu Yi-ren, trans. by Yang Shou-zhong, Blue Poppy Press, Boulder, CO, 1997

General Index

T

tapeworms 133

taxation heat 42, 151, 234

tearing, profuse 14, 20

tenesmus 31, 32, 47, 116, 117, 120, 134

testicular sagging, one-sided 114

testicular swelling and pain 65, 124, 126

tetanus 6, 19, 61, 182, 183, 187

tetany 6, 18, 19, 60, 175, 176, 181-183, 187, 189

tetany reversal 189

thirst, vexatious 15, 25, 44, 53, 64, 65, 72, 73, 99, 140, 224

throat, dry 16, 66, 229

throat, dryness of the nose and 14

throat, inhibited 46

throat pain 62, 78

throat, sore, swollen 18, 20

throat swelling and pain 13, 38, 43-46, 169, 177, 185, 190, 191, 202

throat, ulcerated 46

thromboangitis 152

tidal heat 25, 32, 41, 54, 55, 217, 228

tinnitus 17, 191, 204, 217, 230

tongue, sores in the mouth and on the 27, 101, 158, 170, 177, 191

tongue, sores on the 21

toothache 8, 10

tremors 176, 178, 181-184

trichomoniasis, vaginal tract 47

tuberculosis, pulmonary 139

U

ulcerated sores with profuse pus 240

ulcers, enduring 162

unconsciousness 79

urinary incontinence 42, 121, 213, 233, 238, 239, 243-245, 247

urinary retention, postpartum 104

urinary strangury, dribbling, astringency, and pain 77, 96, 185

urinary tract astringency and pain 158

urinary tract infections 32

urination, astringent, painful 29, 32, 34, 49

urination, difficult 99

urination, frequent 20, 108, 110, 121, 201, 205-209, 213, 233, 238, 243-245, 247

urination, inhibited 4, 69, 73, 79, 84, 93-96, 108, 122, 152, 158, 211, 238

urination, reddish, scanty 27, 29

urination, scanty 27, 29, 69, 101, 102, 198

urination, short, reddish 12, 23, 26, 96, 98, 103

urine, turbid 94

urticaria 18, 167

uterine prolapse 17, 21, 117, 197

V

vacuity vexation 170, 171, 225, 235, 237

vaginal discharge, abnormal 7, 8, 21, 32, 34, 52, 54, 94, 95, 100, 102-104, 113, 142, 178, 179, 201, 205, 210, 233, 240, 243, 248

vaginal tract trichomoniasis 47

vertex, pain at the 10

vertigo 60, 144, 175-178, 181, 182, 186, 218, 226, 227, 238

vexation 20, 23-28, 30, 31, 35, 36, 38, 45, 52, 65, 67, 96, 101, 151, 154, 170, 171, 177, 178, 184, 221, 223, 225, 235, 237

vexation and agitation 23, 24, 26, 30, 31, 35, 36, 38, 45, 65, 177, 178, 184

vision, blurred 14-15, 20, 28, 180, 210, 217, 218, 226, 230

vision, dimmed 96

vision, internal obstruction of 96

visual acuity, decreased 210, 224

visual obstruction, external 35

voice, hoarse 18, 62

vomiting 9, 11, 26, 28, 31, 54, 57-59, 65, 71, 72, 79, 86, 89-92, 107, 109, 112-115, 119, 121, 124-127, 134, 146, 147, 180, 194, 203, 221, 236, 239, 242

vomiting, burping and 180

vomiting and spitting 58, 59, 72, 90, 91, 107, 112, 125, 134, 203, 242

W

walk or stand, inability to 83

wasting and thirsting 15, 25, 37, 56, 64, 194, 198, 201, 217, 226, 229, 235, 236

water swelling 1, 2, 4, 11, 34, 65, 75, 78-81, 83, 84, 88, 93-96, 101, 104, 105, 122, 134, 140, 152, 153, 160, 199, 203

white turbidity 243, 246

whole body joint heaviness, soreness, and pain 84

whole body, face, and eyes superficial edema 69

wind and cold, slight aversion to 44, 84

wind, slight aversion to 20, 44, 84, 99

wind cold damp impediment 3, 6, 7, 83, 89, 205

wind damp impediment pain 1, 60, 87, 88, 150, 159, 162, 173, 182, 183, 214, 216

wind damp impediment pain, soreness, and numbness 87

wind stroke 11, 176, 183, 187, 189, 190, 192, 198

wind stroke phlegm reversal 189, 190, 192

withdrawal 177, 191, 192

worm accumulation abdominal pain 123

worms 34, 52, 72, 80, 103, 112, 123, 133-135, 167

Y

yellowing of the body and eyes 98

Latin Medicinal Index

Pin Yin Medicinal Index

Formula Index

OTHER BOOKS ON CHINESE MEDICINE
AVAILABLE FROM BLUE POPPY PRESS
3450 Penrose Place, Suite 110, Boulder, CO 80301
For ordering 1-800-487-9296 PH. 303\447-8372 FAX 303\245-8362

A NEW AMERICAN ACUPUNCTURE by Mark Seem, ISBN 0-936185-44-9

ACUPOINT POCKET REFERENCE ISBN 0-936185-93-7

ACUPUNCTURE AND MOXIBUSTION FORMULAS & TREATMENTS by Cheng Dan-an, trans. by Wu Ming, ISBN 0-936185-68-6

ACUTE ABDOMINAL SYNDROMES: Their Diagnosis & Treatment by Combined Chinese-Western Medicine by Alon Marcus, ISBN 0-936185-31-7

AGING & BLOOD STASIS: A New Approach to TCM Geriatrics by Yan De-xin, ISBN 0-936185-63-5

AIDS & ITS TREATMENT ACCORDING TO TRADITIONAL CHINESE MEDICINE by Huang Bing-shan, trans. by Fu-Di & Bob Flaws, ISBN 0-936185-28-7

BETTER BREAST HEALTH NATURALLY with CHINESE MEDICINE by Honora Lee Wolfe & Bob Flaws ISBN 0-936185-90-2

THE BOOK OF JOOK: Chinese Medicinal Porridges, An Alternative to the Typical Western Break- fast by B. Flaws, ISBN0-936185-60-0

CHINESE MEDICAL PALMISTRY: Your Health in Your Hand by Zong Xiao-fan & Gary Liscum, ISBN 0-936185-64-3

CHINESE MEDICINAL TEAS: Simple, Proven, Folk Formulas for Common Diseases & Promoting Health by Zong Xiao-fan & Gary Liscum, ISBN 0-936185-76-7

CHINESE MEDICINAL WINES & ELIXIRS by Bob Flaws, ISBN 0-936185-58-9

CHINESE PEDIATRIC MASSAGE THERAPY: *A Parent's & Practitioner's Guide to the Prevention & Treatment of Childhood Illness* by Fan Ya-li, ISBN 0-936185-54-6

CHINESE SELF-MASSAGE THERAPY: The Easy Way to Health by Fan Ya-li ISBN 0-936185-74-0

A COMPENDIUM OF TCM PATTERNS & TREATMENTS by Bob Flaws & Daniel Finney, ISBN 0-936185-70-8

CURING ARTHRITIS NATURALLY WITH CHINESE MEDICINE by Douglas Frank & Bob Flaws ISBN 0-936185-87-2

CURING DEPRESSION NATURALLY WITH CHINESE MEDICINE by Rosa Schnyer & Bob Flaws ISBN 0-936185-94-5

CURING HAY FEVER NATURALLY WITH CHINESE MEDICINE by Bob Flaws, ISBN 0-936185-91-0

CURING HEADACHES NATURALLY WITH CHINESE MEDICINE, by Bob Flaws, ISBN 0-936185-95-3

CURING INSOMNIA NATURALLY WITH CHINESE MEDICINE by Bob Flaws ISBN 0-936185-85-6

CURING PMS NATURALLY WITH CHINESE MEDICINE by Bob Flaws ISBN 0-936185-85-6

THE DAO OF INCREASING LONGEVITY AND CONSERVING ONE'S LIFE by Anna Lin & Bob Flaws, ISBN 0-936185-24-4

THE DIVINE FARMER'S MATERIA MEDICA (*A Translation of the Shen Nong Ben Cao*) by Yang Shou-zhong ISBN 0-936185-96-1

THE DIVINELY RESPONDING CLASSIC: *A Translation of the Shen Ying Jing from Zhen Jiu Da Cheng*, trans. by Yang Shou-zhong & Liu Feng-ting ISBN 0-936185-55-4

DUI YAO: THE ART OF COMBINING CHINESE HERBAL MEDICINALS by Philippe Sionneau ISBN 0-936185-81-3